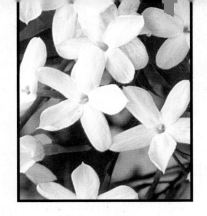

AROMA THERAPY

KATHI KEVILLE

Publications International, Ltd.

Kathi Keville is director of the American Herb Association and editor of the *American Herb Association Quarterly* newsletter. A writer, photographer, consultant, and teacher specializing in aromatherapy and herbs for over 25 years, she has written several books, including *Aromatherapy: The Complete Guide to the Healing Art* and *Pocket Guide to Aromatherapy,* and has written over 150 articles for such magazines as *New Age Journal, The Herb Companion,* and *New Herbal Remedies.*

The author wishes to thank Mary Greer for her editorial assistance on this book.

ACKNOWLEDGMENTS: Excerpt on page 22 from *The Book of Incense: Enjoying Traditional Art of Japanese Scents* by Kiyoko Morita. Published by Kodansha International, Ltd. English translation copyright © 1992 by Kodansha International Ltd. Reprinted by permission. All rights reserved.

PHOTO CREDITS: Front & back cover: **Derek Fell; Steven Foster; Kathi Keville; Ivan Massar/Positive Images; Richard Shiell; Lee Anne White.**

Heather Angel Photography: 33 (top right), 118, 130, 142, 165 (top left); **Cathy Wilkinson Barash:** 107, 149, 165 (right center); **Corbis-Bettmann:** 6 (top left & bottom left), 10, 14, 16, 24, 46 (right center); **Alan & Linda Detrick:** 33 (bottom right), 58 (top right), 93 (top right center), 103, 154, 165 (bottom left); **Derek Fell:** 33 (bottom center), 93 (bottom right center), 144; **Steven Foster:** 93 (top left center, bottom center & bottom right), 105, 109, 135, 140, 163, 165 (top left center & bottom right); **FPG International:** Jim Cummins: 58 (bottom left); Dennis Hallinan: 37; Thomas Lindley: 33 (bottom left); Art Montes de Oca: Table of contents, 46 (bottom right); R. Pleasant: 58 (bottom right center); G. Randall: 33 (right center), 41; Telegraph Colour Library: 33 (top left); **Mindy Green:** 46 (top left, top left center, bottom left center), 48, 58 (bottom right), 70 (left center, bottom right center); **Sam Griffith Studios:** 58 (top left, top right center), 70 (top left & top right, bottom left center), 165 (bottom left center); **Kathi Keville:** 93 (top left & top right), 94, 99, 111, 121, 147, 156, 158; **Erich Lessing/Louvre, Paris/Art Resource:** 6 (top center); **Positive Images:** Karen Bussolini: 101; Ivan Massar: 93 (bottom left center), 128; **Ann Ronan Picture Library:** 46 (top right & bottom left); **Peter Ross Photographs:** 70 (top right center & bottom right); **Richard Shiell:** Title page, 58 (left center), 70 (top center & top left center), 93 (bottom left), 96, 116, 126, 132, 152, 160, 165 (top right); **Carol Simowitz:** 70 (bottom center), 93 (top center), 123; **SuperStock:** 6 (top right & left center), 12; Christie's Images: 6 (bottom right); Musee du Louvre, Paris/Giraudon: 6 (top right center); Stock Montage: 6 (bottom right center); **Lee Anne White:** 33 (left center), 70 (bottom left), 138.

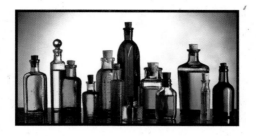

Contents

Introduction

Aroma means scent, and therapy means treatment. Aromatherapy, then, is the use of the fragrant parts of aromatic plants to improve your health and general well-being. First, of course, aromatherapy offers pure enjoyment. Taking a whiff of a spice in your kitchen or a bouquet of flowers is fundamental aromatherapy.

Aromatherapy has many other benefits, too. Inhaling the appropriate fragrance can reduce stress, lift a depression, hasten a good night's sleep, soothe your soul, or give you more energy. Aromatherapy is already helping office workers stay alert while doing repetitive mental tasks. And hospitals are experimenting with using aromatherapy to help patients relax so that other healing modalities can do their job.

Massaging aromatic oils into your skin is another way to benefit from aromatherapy. That's because essential oils, the compounds responsible for a plant's fragrance, offer a multitude of healing benefits in addition to their individual scents. A pungent liniment such as Chinese Tiger Balm, for instance, eases aches and pains. And the latest fragrant shampoos and body oils will improve the health of your complexion and hair while at the same time inducing a particular mood. Aromatherapy, then, is very versatile and can be used in many different ways to treat a wide range of physical and emotional problems.

Many familiar plants provide us with multifaceted essential oils. Rosemary, lavender, orange, and lemon, for example, all produce essential oils that can be used therapeutically. Essential oils from these and other familiar plants are profiled and are used in therapeutic recipes throughout this book.

Aromatherapy: Healing for the Body and Soul covers the basics of aromatherapy. It explains the science behind essential oils—how they influence your emotions and heal physical ailments. And it gives you all the tools you need to begin practicing aromatherapy yourself. You'll learn how to make basic healing applications, such as compresses and gargles, and you'll also find specific recipes to treat a wide variety of conditions, from acne to insomnia to warts.

This book isn't just a how-to on aromatherapy; it also offers a look at the history of aromatherapy through myths, folklore, and traditional uses of the oils and fragrances of aromatic plants. Your interest in aromatherapy makes you part of a long line of people fascinated by the bouquet of nature's odors. You will soon be creating beauty formulas similar to those made for Helen of Troy, Cleopatra, and France's Empress Josephine, as well as healing preparations used by the ancient Greeks, Egyptians, and many other civilizations.

Aromatherapy is so easy to use! Who wouldn't welcome a prescription to bathe with scented oils or to receive an aromatic massage? The simple descriptions in this book will help you put aromatherapy to work enhancing your life.

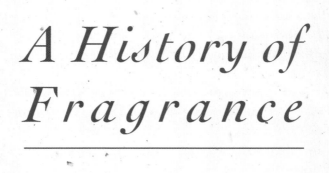

A History of Fragrance

The burning of fragrant woods, leaves, needles, and tree gums as incense is thought to be the earliest form of aromatherapy. This practice probably arose from the discovery that some firewoods, such as cypress and cedar, filled the air with scent when they burned. In fact, our modern word *perfume* is derived from the Latin *per fumum*, which means "through smoke."

Incense was not the only early use of fragrance, however. Sometime between 7000 and 4000 B.C.E., Neolithic tribes learned that animal fats, when heated, absorbed plants' aromatic and healing properties. Perhaps fragrant leaves or flowers accidentally dropped into fat as meat cooked over the fire. The information gleaned from that accident led to other discoveries: Such plants added flavor to food, helped heal wounds, and smoothed dry skin far better than nonscented fat: These fragrant fats — the forerunners of our modern massage and body lotions — scented the wearer, protected skin and hair from weather and insects, and relaxed aching muscles. They also affected people's energies and emotions.

Aromatic water, a third type of fragrant product, was actually a combination of essential oils, water, and alcohol. It was used to enhance the complexion and scent the skin and hair. It also was ingested as a medicinal tonic. It was the forerunner of our modern perfume.

As civilization became more advanced, incense, body oils, and aromatic waters were combined into blends to heal the mind, body, and spirit. Thus, throughout the world, aroma became an integral part of healing and lay the foundation for our use of aromatherapy today.

The Fragrance Trade

In ancient times, as now, commonly used essential oils such as frankincense, eucalyptus, ginger, patchouli, and rosewood came from the furthest reaches of the globe. These vital components of religious ceremonies, medicine, food, cosmetics, and aphrodisiacs were in great demand and were more costly than precious metals and jewels. Although each region could produce clothing, shelter, and food from the resources in its immediate territory, people of all nations craved rare, exotic odors that literally added spice to their lives and lent an air of mystery to their ceremonies.

The demand for aromatic materials, coupled with their portability, led to the establishment of long distance trade. Fortunately, seeds and herbs could be dried, gums rolled into beads, and fragrances infused in oil or solid perfumes while retaining or even improving their properties. This made them extremely portable and relatively impervious to damage.

With trade and the passion for fragrance came adventure and intrigue. Fleets of ships crossed oceans, explorers risked their lives traveling across vast deserts, wars were ignited over land disputes and trade rights, kingdoms were conquered or lost, and love bloomed—all in the pursuit of fragrance. As a result, the quest for fragrance was responsible for molding early world history more than any other single factor.

Babylonian Beginnings

No one knows exactly when trade began, but an import order for cedarwood, myrrh, and cypress was found inscribed on an early Babylonian clay tablet. More than 5,000 years ago, when Egyptians were just learning to write and make bricks, they were already bringing in large quantities of myrrh—their most valued trade import. Certainly there were trade routes through the Middle East to obtain myrrh and other fragrant goods before 2000 B.C.E., and these routes were well-traveled for the next 30 centuries.

Overland trade meant grueling months or even years crossing arid deserts and negotiating difficult mountain passes while being threatened by bandits. So aromatics were soon transported by sea, leading to improvements in sailing techniques, vessels, and navigation. Monsoon winds carried double-outrigger canoes along the cinnamon route through the South Seas. Later, Egyptian and eventually Roman traders took advantage of these same winds to take them to India in the summer and home again in the winter.

The Scent of Royalty

Wheeling and dealing is not a new art, but it was fully employed in the ancient fragrance trade. The great Egyptian Queen Hatshepsut, for one, knew a business opportunity when she saw one. As one of her greatest accomplishments, she sent an expedition to Punt on the African coast to establish what would be a very profitable trade. She also brought back 31 myrrh trees to Egypt, and they were planted in a botanical garden that lined the walkway leading to her massive temple of Deir al-Bahari near Thebes. On the temple walls, the images of the myrrh trees carved in bas-relief can still be seen today.

Other queens made an equal impact on aromatic history. When the Queen of Sheba paid her famous visit to the court of Israel's King Solo-

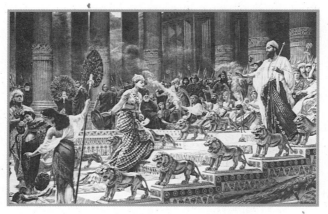

The Queen of Sheba visits King Solomon.

mon, it was to discuss the fragrance trade. Some sources say she was from southwestern Arabia, the land of frankincense and myrrh, but more likely she was queen of a North Arabian tribe that traded the fragrant terebinth resin from the pistachio tree.

Sometimes fragrance simply tagged along in the footsteps of the famous. For example, Alexander the Great's conquests had little to do with the pursuit of fragrant materials. In fact, he despised fragrances because they reminded him of his Persian enemies, and he contemptuously threw out a box of priceless ointments from King Darius' tent after defeating him at the battle of Issos. However, after a few years of traveling through Asia, he became convinced of the joys of fine scent. He anointed his body with fragrant oils and kept incense burning by his throne. And, in his wake, he left the lands he conquered desiring more aromatics.

A World Market

Today, cities prosper and fail with the price of oil. So, too, did they in ancient times; however, it was fragrant oils and spices, not fuel oil, that sparked the growth of key cities along the avenues of commerce. With the introduction of camels as pack animals, the city of Alexandria developed into an active trading hub linking several trade routes, including one to Arabia, 2,000 miles away.

By the fourth century B.C.E., Babylon had a thriving market, trading in cedar of Lebanon, cypress, pine, fir resin, myrtle, calamus, and juniper. Athens was famous for its hundreds of shops selling scented body oils and solid incense/perfumes. Phoenician merchants dealt in Chinese camphor, Indian cinnamon, black pepper, and sandalwood. Africa, South Arabia, and India supplied lemongrass, ginger, and spikenard, the rhizome of which has an exotic fragrance. China imported jasmine-scented sesame oil from India and Persia, rose water via the Silk Route, and eventually, Indonesian aromat-

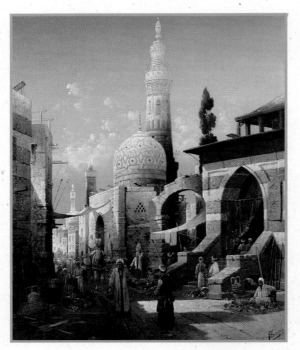

Spices and scented oils were sold in ancient markets.

ics: cloves, gum benzoin, ginger, nutmeg, and patchouli. Astute traders knew which locales produced the best oils and fragrances.

Redolent Wealth

Since ancient times, the wealthy and powerful have been able to drown themselves in fragrance. In fact, one unfortunate Roman literally did. He was asphyxiated when the carved ivory ceiling panels in Emperor Nero's dining room slid aside to shower guests, who reclined on floor pillows, with hundreds of pounds of fresh rose petals. In general, wealthy Romans so overindulged themselves in fragrance that the ruler Leptadeni, in 188 B.C.E., issued an edict forbidding such foolish excess.

The Roman population paid little heed to the fragrance prohibition, and demand for incense only increased. By the first century C.E., Romans were burning 2,800 tons of imported frankincense and 550 tons of myrrh—both herbs more costly than gold—each year. As a result, Emperor Augustus increased the number of trade ships sailing between Egypt and India fivefold, from twenty to a hundred.

Islamic culture was also rich in fragrance, using it extensively in medicine, cosmetics, and confections. Rose water was mixed into the mortar used to build mosques, and even the ground in paradise was said to emit the scent of musk and saffron. Mohammed himself was once a spice and aromatics merchant who traveled on camel caravans. He loved fragrance, especially rose, mentioning it frequently in his teachings: "Whoever would smell my scent, let him smell the rose."

Linking East and West

Although certainly not the intention, the Crusades of the eleventh, twelfth, and thirteenth centuries acquainted the European population with Arabian ideas and fostered an appreciation of Eastern aromatics, despite repeated warnings by the Christian priesthood that fragrance was associated with Satan. Crusaders returned bearing gifts of oils, fragrant waters, and solid perfumes. Soon the European elite were demanding rose water, and Italians could not live without the addition of orange water to their sweets and confections.

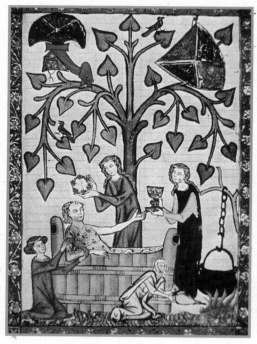

A knight returned from war is treated to a rose bath.

As commerce in fragrance increased between East and West, so did the exchange of ideas. To facilitate trade the Chinese adopted the Indian system of counting. By the eleventh century, Arabs were navigating spice-laden ships from India to China with the Chinese compass and balanced stern rudder. During the next century,

the Chinese navy grew from 3,000 to 50,000 sailors to accommodate large vessels that each hauled as much as six thousand baskets of fragrant herbs and spices.

China's upper classes were lavish in their use of scent, especially from the seventh century T'ang Dynasty through the Ming Dynasty in the seventeenth century. Everything was scented — baths, clothing, buildings, ink, and paper. Miniature landscapes, in which perfumed smoke escaped from a mountain and coiled around the peak, became the rage.

Exploration and Colonization

Marco Polo made his famous journey to Kublai Khan's court in the late thirteenth century to establish direct trade between Italy and China. The Italians could thus circumvent Muslim middlemen and their 300 percent markup. The deal was successful, and throughout the thirteenth and fourteenth century Italy monopolized Eastern trade with Europe. Not to be outdone, Spain sent Christopher Columbus across the ocean to seek a shorter route to India.

It was the Portuguese who established a sailing route to India that circumvented Alexandria and Constantinople. In 1498, Vasco de Gama's sailors cheered, "For Christ and spices!" as they reached India, land of fragrant spices and herbs. They brought back so much that nutmegs were said to be rolling in the streets of Lisbon!

Early in the seventeenth century the Dutch built forts in India, establishing the Dutch East India Company by force. In provinces where they couldn't obtain control, they simply up-

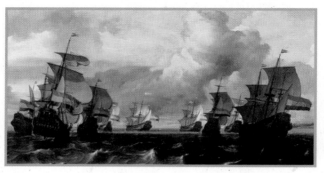

A fleet from the Dutch East India Company sets sail.

rooted nutmeg and clove trees so no one else could have them. But the French managed to slip several fragrant plants out from under the Dutch noses. These were planted in the French West Indies and the island of Bourbon (now called Réunion).

Incense & Solid Perfumes

For thousands of years and throughout the world, fragrant smoke has purified the air and comforted individuals who were in physical, emotional, or spiritual need. At first, tossing a few fragrant plant twigs into the fire served the purpose, but eventually solid incense was created using ground gums and plants mixed with honey. These were formed into solid cubes and set on a coal from the fire. In many cultures, elaborate ceremonial burners were designed to hold cubes of incense atop smoldering coals.

Purification

The ancients filled temples, council rooms, and homes with incense, using it even more liberally than we would an air freshner. Small wonder, since incense was able to dispel the disagreeable smells of unsanitary living conditions. In Europe, Arabia, India, China, and throughout North America, dwellings were fumigated to drive out the evil spirits that were believed to cause illness while, at the same time, ridding the dwelling of fleas and bugs. During epidemics, people who flocked to temples and churches were probably helped by the burning of antiseptic herbs. Hippocrates, the father of medicine, is said to have freed Athens from the plague by burning aromatic plants, as did Moses and Aaron in the desert (Num 16;46–50).

Respiratory and rheumatic ills, headaches, unconsciousness, and other medical problems were treated by breathing in smoke arising from aromatic plants. And sometimes wet, aromatic herbs or herb teas were dropped on hot rocks to create a steam that was inhaled. Both techniques proved effective in treating sinus congestion, lung problems, or earache.

During religious and healing ceremonies, Native Americans burned tight bundles of fragrant herbs and braids of the vanillalike sweet grass and surrounded themselves in the smoke. And to heal the sick, rocks steaming from the tea of goldenrod, fleabane, pearly everlasting, and echinacea were placed next to a patient, and both were covered with hides or blankets to make a type of aroma-filled mini-sauna.

Versatile Arómata

Throughout Europe, Arabia, and India, incense proved to be immensely versatile; it was used as perfume, medicine, and even mouthwash. Remember, early incense contained nothing other than ground herbs, plant gums, and honey. (Only much later was messy charcoal and inedible saltpeter added so that, once ignited, it would continue burning.) Since most of the herbs were highly antiseptic, when rubbed on the skin and melted by body heat, they released a scent and disinfected wounds. Incense was even ingested as medicine. It is no surprise, then, that the Greek word *arómata* had several meanings: incense, perfume, spice, and aromatic medicine. The Chinese also had one word, *heang,* to describe perfume, incense, and the concept of fragrance.

Some aromatics were even found to help with weight loss, digestion, or menstrual regularity. Rome's most famous perfume, Susinon, when ingested was a diuretic and relieved various types of inflammation. Amarakinon treated indigestion and hemorrhoids and encouraged menstruation, either when ingested or applied directly to the affliction. It was also worn as perfume. Spikenard was the main ingredient in another perfume that could be sucked as a throat lozenge to relieve coughs and laryngitis.

An Intoxication of Mind and Emotions

Throughout the world, incense has been employed to affect mind and emotions. According to the Japanese, it fosters communication with the transcendent, purifies mind and body, keeps you alert, acts as a companion in the midst of solitude, and brings moments of peace amidst busy affairs. The fragrant smoke billowing from Chinese bronze incense burners was classified into six basic moods: tranquil, reclusive, luxurious, beautiful, refined, and noble.

Certain plants have been burned for their intoxicating or aphrodisiac properties. In Delphi, Greece, the oracle priestesses sat on stools over holes in the floor that emitted fumes of bay leaves to inspire visions. While little of Delphi's grandeur remains today, you can still see the hidden incense chamber underneath the floor. Women in Tibet called *dainyals* held cloths over their heads to capture cedar smoke, which would send them into prophetic chanting. Aromatic plants with hypnotic properties were used similarly by Australian aborigines and by Native Americans.

Cleopatra used the bewitchment of scent to lure Mark Anthony. Her slaves fanned smoke from burning incense onto the sails of her ship. In *Anthony and Cleopatra*, Shakespeare describes these sails as "so perfumed that the winds were lovesick with them." This was probably not far from the truth, since the scent she chose is thought to be that of the delicious camphire (henna) mentioned in the Song of Solomon — long regarded as an aphrodisiac.

Religious Uses of Incense

In nearly every culture, incense was believed to attract the gods and goddesses, keep evil spirits at bay, and purify both body and soul. Ancient peoples, believing that spirit and life entered the body through their breath, also thought that inhaling certain odors brought them closer to God. Fragrance was considered akin to the divine because it was invisible, mysterious, and attractive. They called aroma the soul of the plant and thought it a gift from God. They also believed that the deities would find prayers — breathed into the smoke which carried them aloft — more pleasing when sweetly scented.

Its association with sensuality and its excessive use by Arabs, Romans, and Jews gave incense a bad name among most early Christians. However, some sects did use it exclusively for religious ceremonies. Gnostic Christians of the first to fourth centuries were deeply influenced by Egyptian philosophy and adopted the ancient belief that a plant's fragrance is associated with the soul of man. Eventually, the Catholic church embraced the use of incense to purify and bless their statues, relics, altars, and those participating in the mass.

To the Chinese Taoist, fragrance also held a religious significance. Among the 10,000 rites of Taoist Buddhism, it is said that the "burning of incense has primacy," representing the soul's liberation from limitations of the material world. To enhance their experience, they sometimes incorporated psychoactive plants such as cannabis into their incense. The incense burner itself, called *fa lu,* became an object of worship.

The Art and Practice of Scent

Although the Japanese came relatively late to the use of incense, they quickly developed it into a sophisticated art called *koh-do* that was taught in special schools. Still practiced by a few people today, participants in the incense ceremony had to bathe and dress in clean clothes so that they carried no odors into the room. They then tried ess the different characteristics of the in- he winner went home with a prize. ese, during the Nara and Kamakura 333 C.E.), were especially practi- o household uses of incense.

A clock changed scent as time passed. A more sophisticated clock announced the time according to which chimney issued smoke. Geisha even kept track of their customer's stay by how many sticks of incense burned. A special headrest called a *kikohmakura* imparted perfumed smoke to a lady's hair, and kimonas were hung on a rack over scented smoke.

The world's first novel, *Prince Genji*, written by Lady Murasaki Shikibu in the eleventh century, describes the practice of scenting one's kimono sleeves. Small incense burners were "held for a moment inside each sleeve" so that scent floated about whenever a motion was made by the hand. Japan's earliest anthology of poems refers to this practice:

In the moonlight
Where are the plum blossoms?
Let their fragrance guide you.
The fragrance —
More alluring than the color —
Whose scented sleeves have brushed
The blossoms in my garden?
— From the *Kokinshu*, 905 C.E.

The European elite also scented their sle
Ladies of the court pinned scented pen
held solid perfumes imported from
the sleeves of their cut-velvet g
kept the perfume in lockets

neck where they could be conveniently sniffed. Orange blossom oil was extracted and combined with pressed almond pulp to make the very popular perfume ointment pomades. *Pomme d'ambre,* on the other hand, were scented balls of ambergris, spices, honey, and wine that hung from the belt in a small, perforated container. Even the slightest movement of a skirt would surround one in fragrance.

Body Oils

Fragrance also found its way into religious and secular life via scented oils. These were made, as they still are today, by extracting plant oils into fat or vegetable oil and then straining out the used plant material. They were used liberally in religious ceremonies to consecrate temples, alters, statues, candles, and priests.

Religious Use of Fragrant Oils

The Book of Exodus (30:22–25) provides one of the earliest recipes for an anointing oil—given by God to Moses to be used in the initiation of priests. The ingredients included myrrh, cinnamon, calamus, and cassia blended into olive oil.

When Mary Magdalene anointed Christ's feet and wiped them with her hair, it was with an oil made from costly spikenard. The name Christ, or Christos, from the Greek *chriein,* literally means

and
tainly

did not enjoy the messy
nd straining scented oils,
rs from Egypt. Men and
bathed in fragrance. So
of scent that Romans af-
r sweethearts "my myrrh,
today we call our loved

pecially attracted to the
fact, Hippocrates recom-
ody oils in the bath. In
f unguentarii shops sold
sage, anise, rose, and iris
ened with beeswax. They
ts (from a word meaning
small, elaborately deco-
they still do today. How-

per-
Gedi, by
parently of-
ts, since the
at are be-
atment
spe-
ok

rance

atherapy
25

"to anoint," and the frankincense and myrrh brought by the wise men to the Christ child most likely were anointing oils. These oils were con-

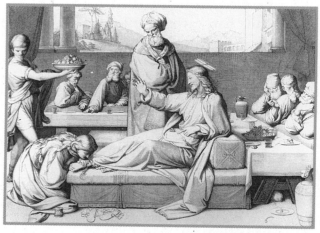

Mary Magdalene anoints Christ's feet with oil.

sidered to be more valuable than the gold that was carried by the third wise man.

Ancient Egyptian Scents

Egyptian talent for formulating scented became legendary, and their oils were ce potent: Calcite pots filled wit still held a faint odor when tomb was opened 3,000 yea were especially creative wi did not restrict it to r ual's special odor, a hieroglyph of of influenci

ever, in those times the shopkeepers were con-sulted as doctors, and their products were sold for a multitude of medicinal uses.

Greek men and women anointed their bodie for both personal enhancement and ser

The men used a different scented its particular attributes, body. Most of the oil the arms, we Oils for games.

East India into a veritable garc anointed themselves with patchouli on the neck and cheek breasts, spikenard in the hair, musk domen, sandalwood on the thighs, and saffro their feet. Men, however, applied only sandal-wood to their own bodies.

The daily bathing ritual in India required the application of sesame oils scented with jasmine, coriander, cardamom, basil, costus, pandanus, agarwood, pine, saffron, champac, and clove. Ancient Vedic religious and medical books gave instruction on balancing body temperature, tem perament, and digestion with such aromas some of their therapeutic uses were ce passed on to the West.

In Egypt, everyone used body oils, from royalty to laborers. Builders constructing a burial site went on strike in the twelfth century B.C.E. not just because the food was bad, but even worse, they complained, "We have no ointment." They depended upon the oils to ease sore muscles after a day of hauling and carving huge stones and to protect their skin from the intense Egyptian sun.

Throughout the Americas, massage with scented oils was also used as therapy and was often the first treatment given. One massage oil prepared by the Incas contained valerian and other relaxing herbs that were thickened with seaweed. The Aztecs massaged the sick with scented ointments in their sweat lodges.

Perfume

Perfume as we know it today—packaged in tiny, expensive bottles with a high alcohol content and hundreds of chemical compounds—is a relatively new invention.

Maria Prophetissa's Invention

The first written description of a distiller to to g͏uce essential oils appears around the first cense. ͏y C.E. Maria Prophetissa, known as Mary The Japan ͏ss, invented a mechanism that looked Periods (710–1 like a double-boiler. She described cal when it came t the essential oil it produced as an "angel who descends from the sky." By the second century C.E. the Chinese and Arabs were distilling essential oils, and Japan followed suit a few centuries later.

Prophetissa's inventions could also distill alcohol. Combining it with essential oils and diluting it with water produced a new type of fragrance. These scented "waters" made the body smell sweet and also acted as medicine and cosmetics. When dabbed on the skin, they improved skin tone and diminished blemishes. When taken internally, they relieved indigestion, soothed menstrual cramps, or treated myriad other ailments. Thus was born the "medicinal tonic."

Aromatic Waters

If you have ever appreciated a fine European liquor such as Benedictine or Fra Angelica, you are benefiting from the stills of early monastery infirmaries and herbariums. Many monks and nuns were dedicated herbalists who served as both doctor and pharmacist to their patients. Aromatic waters were one of their favorite prescriptions.

Some sources credit the twelfth century herbalist Saint Hildegard, Abbess of Bingen, with inventing lavender water, which she mentions in a treatise on medicinal and aromatic herbs. However it originated, this aromatic water took Europe by storm. By the fourteenth century, lavender water was so popular that the French King Charles V had lavender planted in the gardens at the Louvre to ensure the supply.

Another famous monastic concoction was *Aqua Mirabilis,* or "Miracle Water," a water and alcohol

---

THE LEGEND OF ROSE OIL

One poetic story credits the discovery of the essential oil of roses to seventeenth century Persian princess Nour-Djihan. During her wedding procession, while she was being rowed in a canal strewn with rose petals, Nour swept her hand through the water. The hot day had caused the oil from the roses to float on the water's surface and her hand emerged covered with perfumed droplets. She convinced her father to have his alchemist learn to extract this essence, and thus began the manufacture of essential oil of roses.

---

combination spiked with essential oils. It was sipped to improve vision and to treat rheumatic pain, fever, and congestion; it was also said to improve memory and reduce melancholy. In addition, it was splashed on the body to improve one's smell. Carmelite Water was prepared by European Carmelite nuns from a secret formula that we now know included melissa (lemon balm) and angelica. It aided both digestion and

the complexion, depending upon its use. Modern versions of Miracle Water and Carmelite
Water are still sold in Europe today.

Eau de Cologne

In 1732, aromatic waters were further refined
into cologne when Giovanni Maria Farina of
Cologne, France, took over his uncle's business.
Aqua Admirabilis, a lively blend of neroli, bergamot, lavender, and rosemary in grape alcohol,
which has a distinct fruity scent, was used on the
face and also treated sore gums and indigestion.
Soldiers dubbed it "Eau de Cologne," meaning
Cologne water, after the town, and the name
cologne stuck to all perfumed waters since then.
The rumor was that Napoleon went through
several bottles a day, an endorsement that made
the cologne so popular that 39 nearly identical
products were created. A half century of lawsuits against these illegal knock-off colognes followed.

After four centuries as the undisputed favorite,
Queen of Hungary Water was displaced by Eau
de Cologne as the fragrance in most demand.

Chemistry and Cosmetics

A little more than 100 years ago, the fragrance
industry was suddenly thrust into the modern
chemical age. Previously, cologne and even soap
had always been considered part of the medici-

gious ceremonies. Gnostic Christians of the first to fourth centuries were deeply influenced by Egyptian philosophy and adopted the ancient belief that a plant's fragrance is associated with the soul of man. Eventually, the Catholic church embraced the use of incense to purify and bless their statues, relics, altars; and those participating in the mass.

To the Chinese Taoist, fragrance also held a religious significance. Among the 10,000 rites of Taoist Buddhism, it is said that the "burning of incense has primacy," representing the soul's liberation from limitations of the material world. To enhance their experience, they sometimes incorporated psychoactive plants such as cannabis into their incense. The incense burner itself, called *fa lu,* became an object of worship.

The Art and Practice of Scent

Although the Japanese came relatively late to the use of incense, they quickly developed it into a sophisticated art called *koh-do* that was taught in special schools. Still practiced by a few people today, participants in the incense ceremony had to bathe and dress in clean clothes so that they carried no odors into the room. They then tried to guess the different characteristics of the incense. The winner went home with a prize.

The Japanese, during the Nara and Kamakura Periods (710–1333 C.E.), were especially practical when it came to household uses of incense.

A clock changed scent as time passed. A more sophisticated clock announced the time according to which chimney issued smoke. Geisha even kept track of their customer's stay by how many sticks of incense burned. A special headrest called a *kikohmakura* imparted perfumed smoke to a lady's hair, and kimonas were hung on a rack over scented smoke.

The world's first novel, *Prince Genji,* written by Lady Murasaki Shikibu in the eleventh century, describes the practice of scenting one's kimono sleeves. Small incense burners were "held for a moment inside each sleeve" so that scent floated about whenever a motion was made by the hand. Japan's earliest anthology of poems refers to this practice:

> In the moonlight
> Where are the plum blossoms?
> Let their fragrance guide you.
> The fragrance—
> More alluring than the color—
> Whose scented sleeves have brushed
> The blossoms in my garden?
> —From the *Kokinshu,* 905 C.E.

The European elite also scented their sleeves. Ladies of the court pinned scented pendants that held solid perfumes imported from Arabia into the sleeves of their cut-velvet gowns. They also kept the perfume in lockets worn around the neck where they could be conveniently sniffed. Orange blossom oil was extracted and combined with pressed almond pulp to make the very popular perfume ointment pomades. *Pomme d'ambre,* on the other hand, were scented balls of ambergris, spices, honey, and wine that hung from the belt in a small, perforated container. Even the slightest movement of a skirt would surround one in fragrance.

Body Oils

Fragrance also found its way into religious and secular life via scented oils. These were made, as they still are today, by extracting plant oils into fat or vegetable oil and then straining out the used plant material. They were used liberally in religious ceremonies to consecrate temples, alters, statues, candles, and priests.

Religious Use of Fragrant Oils

The Book of Exodus (30:22–25) provides one of the earliest recipes for an anointing oil—given by God to Moses to be used in the initiation of priests. The ingredients included myrrh, cinnamon, calamus, and cassia blended into olive oil.

When Mary Magdalene anointed Christ's feet and wiped them with her hair, it was with an oil made from costly spikenard. The name Christ, or Christos, from the Greek *chriein,* literally means "to anoint," and the frankincense and myrrh brought by the wise men to the Christ child most likely were anointing oils. These oils were con-

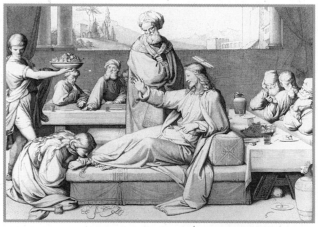

Mary Magdalene anoints Christ's feet with oil.

sidered to be more valuable than the gold that was carried by the third wise man.

Ancient Egyptian Scents

Egyptian talent for formulating scented oils became legendary, and their oils were certainly potent: Calcite pots filled with richly scented oils still held a faint odor when King Tutankamen's tomb was opened 3,000 years later. Egyptians were especially creative with the use of scent and did not restrict it to religious rites. An individual's special odor, or *khaibt*, was represented by a hieroglyph of a fan and was thought capable of influencing the emotions of others.

The first beauty spa may have been the perfume factory owned by Cleopatra at En Gedi, by the Dead Sea. Individuals were apparently offered health and beauty treatments, since the ruins of the factory show seats in what are believed to have been waiting and treatment rooms. Fragrant herbs were blended into specially prepared olive oil. Unfortunately, the book in which Cleopatra recorded recipes for her body oils, *Cleopatra Gynaeciarum Libri,* is long lost. We know of it only through its mention in Roman texts.

Bathed in Fragrance

The Romans, who did not enjoy the messy process of infusing and straining scented oils, imported most of theirs from Egypt. Men and women alike literally bathed in fragrance. So prevalent was the use of scent that Romans affectionately called their sweethearts "my myrrh, my cinnamon," just as today we call our loved ones "honey."

The Greeks were especially attracted to the use of scented oils. In fact, Hippocrates recommended the use of body oils in the bath. In Athens, proprietors of unguentarii shops sold marjoram, lily, thyme, sage, anise, rose, and iris infused in oil and thickened with beeswax. They packaged their unguents (from a word meaning to smear or anoint) in small, elaborately decorated ceramic pots, as they still do today. How-

ever, in those times the shopkeepers were con-
sulted as doctors, and their products were sold
for a multitude of medicinal uses.

Greek men and women anointed their bodies
for both personal enhancement and sensuality.
The men used a different scented oil, chosen for
its particular attributes, for each part of their
body. Most of the oils they used, such as mint for
the arms, were warm and stimulating.

Oils were also used to massage tight muscles.
Athletes in India, on the Mediterranean island of
Crete, and later in Greece and Rome, had specially prepared oils rubbed into their muscles before, and often after, participating in their athletic
games.

East Indian Tantric practice turned women
into a veritable garden of earthly delights. They
anointed themselves with jasmine on their hands,
patchouli on the neck and cheeks, amber on their
breasts, spikenard in the hair, musk on the abdomen, sandalwood on the thighs, and saffron on
their feet. Men, however, applied only sandalwood to their own bodies.

The daily bathing ritual in India required the
application of sesame oils scented with jasmine,
coriander, cardamom, basil, costus, pandanus,
agarwood, pine, saffron, champac, and clove.
Ancient Vedic religious and medical books gave
instruction on balancing body temperature, tem-
perament, and digestion with such aromas, and
some of their therapeutic uses were certainly
passed on to the West.

In Egypt, everyone used body oils, from royalty to laborers. Builders constructing a burial site went on strike in the twelfth century B.C.E. not just because the food was bad, but even worse, they complained, "We have no ointment." They depended upon the oils to ease sore muscles after a day of hauling and carving huge stones and to protect their skin from the intense Egyptian sun.

Throughout the Americas, massage with scented oils was also used as therapy and was often the first treatment given. One massage oil prepared by the Incas contained valerian and other relaxing herbs that were thickened with seaweed. The Aztecs massaged the sick with scented ointments in their sweat lodges.

Perfume

Perfume as we know it today—packaged in tiny, expensive bottles with a high alcohol content and hundreds of chemical compounds—is a relatively new invention.

Maria Prophetissa's Invention

The first written description of a distiller to produce essential oils appears around the first century C.E. Maria Prophetissa, known as Mary the Jewess, invented a mechanism that looked something like a double-boiler. She described

the essential oil it produced as an "angel who descends from the sky." By the second century C.E.
the Chinese and Arabs were distilling essential
oils, and Japan followed suit a few centuries
later.

Prophetissa's inventions could also distill alcohol. Combining it with essential oils and diluting
it with water produced a new type of fragrance.
These scented "waters" made the body smell
sweet and also acted as medicine and cosmetics.
When dabbed on the skin, they improved skin
tone and diminished blemishes. When taken internally, they relieved indigestion, soothed menstrual cramps, or treated myriad other ailments.
Thus was born the "medicinal tonic."

Aromatic Waters

If you have ever appreciated a fine European
liquor such as Benedictine or Fra Angelica, you
are benefiting from the stills of early monastery
infirmaries and herbariums. Many monks and
nuns were dedicated herbalists who served as
both doctor and pharmacist to their patients.
Aromatic waters were one of their favorite prescriptions.

Some sources credit the twelfth century
herbalist Saint Hildegard, Abbess of Bingen,
with inventing lavender water, which she mentions in a treatise on medicinal and aromatic
herbs. However it originated, this aromatic
water took Europe by storm. By the fourteenth

century, lavender water was so popular that the French King Charles V had lavender planted in the gardens at the Louvre to ensure the supply.

Another famous monastic concoction was *Aqua Mirabilis,* or "Miracle Water," a water and alcohol

THE LEGEND OF ROSE OIL

One poetic story credits the discovery of the essential oil of roses to seventeenth century Persian princess Nour-Djihan. During her wedding procession, while she was being rowed in a canal strewn with rose petals, Nour swept her hand through the water. The hot day had caused the oil from the roses to float on the water's surface and her hand emerged covered with perfumed droplets. She convinced her father to have his alchemist learn to extract this essence, and thus began the manufacture of essential oil of roses.

combination spiked with essential oils. It was sipped to improve vision and to treat rheumatic pain, fever, and congestion; it was also said to improve memory and reduce melancholy. In addition, it was splashed on the body to improve one's smell. Carmelite Water was prepared by European Carmelite nuns from a secret formula that we now know included melissa (lemon balm) and angelica. It aided both digestion and the complexion, depending upon its use. Modern versions of Miracle Water and Carmelite Water are still sold in Europe today.

Eau de Cologne

In 1732, aromatic waters were further refined into cologne when Giovanni Maria Farina of Cologne, France, took over his uncle's business. *Aqua Admirabilis,* a lively blend of neroli, bergamot, lavender, and rosemary in grape alcohol, which has a distinct fruity scent, was used on the face and also treated sore gums and indigestion. Soldiers dubbed it "Eau de Cologne," meaning Cologne water, after the town, and the name cologne stuck to all perfumed waters since then. The rumor was that Napoleon went through several bottles a day, an endorsement that made the cologne so popular that 39 nearly identical products were created. A half century of lawsuits against these illegal knock-off colognes followed.

After four centuries as the undisputed favorite, Queen of Hungary Water was displaced by Eau de Cologne as the fragrance in most demand.

Chemistry and Cosmetics

A little more than 100 years ago, the fragrance industry was suddenly thrust into the modern chemical age. Previously, cologne and even soap had always been considered part of the medici-

nal pharmacy. Then, in 1867, the Paris International Exhibition boldly exhibited them in a separate section dubbed cosmetics. This radical move birthed an entirely new industry that paved the way for a new product: perfume.

The very next year, the first commercial synthetic essential oil was developed in the laboratory. With its fresh smell of newly mowed hay, the synthetic oil was an instant hit with cologne manufacturers. Thousands of synthetic fragrances, even those imitating the rarest and most expensive essential oils, were engineered mostly from petroleum chemicals.

These synthetic oils changed the character of personal fragrance forever. The new chemicals were so concentrated, they allowed the manufacture of powerful perfumes. Replacing light colognes that were liberally splashed on, just a few small drops of perfume completely scented an individual. Still other newly-invented chemical additives made that scent linger for hours. Of course, with all the synthetic ingredients, colognes and perfumes were no longer medicinal—and certainly not edible. For the first time in history, they were purely a cosmetic product.

Promoted by the newly emerging fashion design world, major perfume houses such as Guerlain, Bourjois, and Rimmel established themselves in France. While the Victorian era had frowned on anything but the lightest scents, styles changed when American soldiers returned from France following World War I, laden with gifts of perfume. The idea of wearing a personal fragrance caught on.

Aromatherapy Comes of Age

Today, perfume, food, medicine, and aromatherapy products are viewed as separate entities, although aromatherapy is slowly reclaiming its medicinal heritage. A French chemist, René-Maurice Gattefossé, coined the term aromatherapie in 1928. His family were perfumers, but his interest in the therapeutic use of essential oils began when he severely burned his hand in a laboratory explosion. He deliberately plunged his hand into a nearby container of lavender oil to ease the pain, but was amazed at how quickly it healed. He wrote numerous books and papers on the chemistry of perfume and cosmetics. Around the same time another Frenchman, Albert Couvreur, published a book on the medicinal uses of essential oils.

A new wave of aromatherapist practitioners was inspired by this work, one of whom was Dr. Jean Valnet, who, while an army surgeon during World War II, used essential oils such as thyme, clove, lemon, and chamomile on wounds and burns. He later used essential oils to treat psychiatric problems. Marguerite Maury, a French biochemist, developed therapeutic methods for applying these oils to the skin as a massage, reintroducing an ancient method of aromatherapy to the modern world.

Healing Benefits

Remember the heady fragrance of an herb or flower garden on a hot summer's day, or the crisp smell of an orange as you peel it? These odors are the fragrance of the plant's essential oils, the potent, volatile, and aromatic substance contained in various parts of the plant, including its flowers, leaves, roots, wood, seeds, fruit, and bark. The essential oils carry concentrations of the plant's healing properties—those same properties that traditional Western medicine utilizes in many drugs.

What is Aromatherapy?

Aromatherapy simply means the application of those healing powers — it is a fragrant cure. Professional aromatherapists focus very specifically on the controlled use of essential oils to treat ailments and disease and to promote physical and emotional well-being.

Aromatherapy doesn't just work through the sense of smell alone, however. Inhalation is only one application method. Essential oils can also be applied to the skin. When used topically, the oils penetrate the skin, taking direct action on body tissues and organs in the vicinity of application. They also enter the bloodstream and are carried throughout the body. Of course, when applied topically the fragrance of the essential oil is also inhaled.

There are three different modes of action in the body: pharmacological, which affects the chemistry of the body; physiological, which affects the ability of the body to function and process; and psychological, which affects emotions and attitudes. These three modes interact continuously. Aromatherapy is so powerful partly because it affects all three modes. You choose the application method based on where you most want the effects concentrated and on what is most convenient and pleasing to you.

Aromatherapy is actually an aspect of a larger category of healing treatment known as herbal medicine. Herbal medicine also utilizes the healing powers of plants to treat physical and emotional problems, but it uses the whole plant or parts of the plant, such as leaves, flowers, roots, and seeds, rather than the essential oil. Aromatherapy and herbal medicine can be used individually, or they can be used jointly to augment potential healing benefits.

Therapeutic Uses of Essential Oils

You can treat a wide range of physical problems with aromatherapy. Almost all essential oils have antiseptic properties and are able to fight infection and destroy bacteria, fungi, yeast, parasites, and/or viruses. Many essential oils also reduce aches and pain, soothe or rout inflammations and spasms, stimulate the immune system and insulin and hormone production, affect blood circulation, dissolve mucus and open nasal passages, or aid digestion — just to mention a few of their amazing properties. For the purposes of this book, we will consider basic beauty care as a therapeutic treatment that helps establish well-being. For instance, using aromatherapy in cosmetics and skin preparations can help counter external problems such as skin infections and eczema. It simply depends on which essential oils you use and how you use them.

Aromatherapy can also have a considerable influence on our emotions. Sniffing clary sage, for example, can quell panic, while the fragrance released by peeling an orange can make you feel more optimistic. Since your mind strongly influences your health and is itself a powerful healing tool, it makes aromatherapy's potential even more exciting.

Many essential oils perform more than one function, so having just a half-dozen or so on hand will help you treat a wide range of common physical ailments and emotional problems. The beauty of aromatherapy is that you can create a blend of oils that will benefit both in one treatment. For example, you can blend a combination of essential oils that not only stops indigestion, but also reduces the nervous condition that encouraged it. Or, you could design an aromatherapy body lotion that both improves your complexion and relieves depression.

The Essence of Essential Oils

Plants take the light of the sun, the minerals of the earth, and the carbon dioxide exhaled by humans and animals and, through photosynthesis, transform them into the building blocks of medicine. Among the most important therapeutic compounds manufactured by plants are essential oils. These volatile oils contain a variety of active constituents and are also responsible for each plant's unique fragrance.

Fragrance Molecules

The basic elements of carbon, hydrogen, and oxygen combine to form the different organic molecular compounds that produce aromas. So far, more than 30,000 of these molecular com-

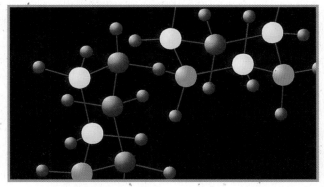

Fragrances consist of many molecular compounds.

pounds have been identified and named. Most individual essential oils consist of many different aromatic molecular compounds. In fact, the essential oil from just one plant may contain as many as one hundred different fragrance molecules. In nature there are thousands of plants, all with unique fragrances that are comprised of different combinations of these molecules.

Plants that smell similar to one another usually contain some of the same molecular compounds. Lemon verbena, lemon balm (melissa), lemon thyme, lemon eucalyptus, citronella, lemongrass, and lemon itself, for instance, all smell like lemon because they contain a lemon-scented molecule called citral. But it is the other aromatic molecules they contain that give each plant its unique fragrance.

Aromatic compounds are grouped under larger classes of compounds such as terpenes, phenols, aldehydes, alcohols, ketones, acids, esters, coumarins, and occasionally, oxides. Citral is an aldehyde; eugenol is a phenol. Each molecular compound has characteristic scents and actions on the body. Some may be cooling and relaxing, while others are warming and stimulating. Some are better for treating indigestion, while others are antiseptic. (See pages 42–43.)

Every effect of an essential oil has a chemical explanation. These effects include their biological activity in the body (beneficial, irritating, or toxic), their solubility (in oil or alcohol, for instance), how rapidly they evaporate in air or are absorbed through the skin, and how well different oils combine as scents. Aldehydes such as those found in cinnamon and lemongrass, for example, have a slightly fruity odor and may often cause skin irritation and allergic reaction. Ketones found in fennel, caraway, and rosemary are not metabolized easily and may pass unchanged into the urine. The phenols found in clove and thyme are very likely to be irritating.

The proportion of aromatic compounds in a particular type of plant is not necessarily constant. This proportion can change from year to year depending on the plants's growing conditions, including geographic location, elevation, climate, soil quality, and the methods used to harvest it and extract the essential oil. Consistent variations found in the same species are called chemotypes, or chemical types (CT). Aromatherapists often take advantage of these natural alterations, selecting a certain chemotype over the standard for its special attributes.

The Physiology of Scent

Essential oil molecules enter the body through the nose and the skin. Since these molecules are extremely small and float easily through the air, you can simply inhale them into your lungs, which then disperse them into your bloodstream. The blood quickly carries them throughout your body. Essential oil molecules are also small enough to be absorbed through the pores of the skin. Once absorbed, some molecules enter the bloodstream, while others remain in the area of application or evaporate into the air. How much goes where depends on the size of the essential oil molecules, the method of application (massage increases absorption), and the carrier containing the essential oil, be it alcohol, vegetable oil, vinegar, or water. This makes essential oils perfect for healing a specific skin problem as well as the entire body.

The sense of smell has its own important mechanisms. High in the nose is the olfactory epithelium, two smell receptors about the size of dimes. The receptors pick up volatile and lipid-soluble molecules using tiny filaments called *cilia*, which may actually be able to identify odor molecules by their "shape." It is believed that these odor receptors are coded by a huge family of genes to sense particular components of smell that produce a characteristic "fingerprint" pattern of activity in the brain.

From the olfactory mucus membrane, signals travel to olfactory bulbs that extend forward like tiny spoons from the brain. An electrical impulse then goes directly to the limbic system, which is part of what is called the primitive or "old" brain. Smell, it seems, was our first sense, and our old brain actually evolved from the olfactory stalks. Because recognition of smell moves directly into the old brain, it completely bypasses areas that control reasoning and the central nervous system. Thus, it directly influences survival mechanisms such as "fight or flight" reactions and the autonomic functions of the body, including heartbeat, body temperature, appetite, digestion, sexual arousal, and memory—the functions we can't control by will or reason. It also affects instincts such as emotions, attraction/repulsion, lust, and creativity. The senses of hearing and vision, by contrast, first stimulate the thalamus, which registers only warmth and pain. Furthermore, the old brain is directly connected to the hypothalamus and pituitary glands, and therefore to our immune system and hormones, which is why smell affects them so powerfully.

Damage to the limbic system of the old brain has been found to adversely affect memory and cause eating disorders and sexual dysfunction. Thus, medical researchers hope to someday treat such memory disorders as Alzheimer disease with fragrance. Other treatments being researched include those for fatigue, migraine headaches, food cravings, depression, schizophrenia, and anxiety.

Essential Oils and Our Daily Lives

Have you ever smelled a certain flower or cologne and suddenly experienced déjà vu? Or

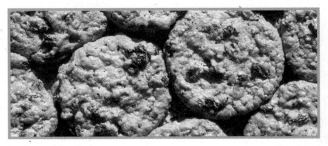

Smelling baking cookies triggers childhood memories.

perhaps you've caught a whiff of fir and immediately envisioned a Christmas tree even in the middle of July. Scent can transport us back to

MEDICINAL PROPERTIES
OF AROMATIC COMPOUNDS

TERPENES AND SESQUITERPENES: antiseptic, anti-inflammatory, carminative, and stimulating. Found in a majority of essential oils, including citruses, flowers, leaves, seeds, roots, and woods. Essential oils in this group: cardamom, carrot seed, cypress, ginger, grapefruit, sandalwood, spikenard, patchouli.

PHENOLS: stimulating, strongly antibacterial, can be skin irritants. Essential oils in this group: clove, oregano, savory, some thymes.

ALDEHYDES: calming, sedating, antiseptic, anti-inflammatory, popular perfume aromatics. Essential oils in this group: cinnamon, cumin, lemon scents.

ALCOHOLS: toning, energizing, antibacterial, antiviral, with pleasant, uplifting fragrances. Essential oils in this group: geranium, rosewood, petitgrain, rose, tea tree.

KETONES: dissolves mucus and fats, heals wounds, includes some toxic factors. Essential oils in this group: sage, hyssop, pennyroyal, jasmine, fennel, peppermint.

ACIDS: anti-inflammatory, antiseptic, moisturizing. Mostly found in combination with alcohols to create esters. Essential oils in this group: birch, rosewood, niaouli.

ESTERS: balancing, relaxing, soothing, antispasmodic, antifungal, with fruity aromas. Essential oils in this group: lavender, bergamot, clary sage, ylang ylang, neroli, Roman chamomile, marjoram.

COUMARINS: calming and uplifting, blood thinning, photosensitizing, some toxic properties. Essential oils in this group: bergamot, angelica, citruses.

OXIDES: expectorant. Essential oils in this group: eucalyptus, bay, hyssop.

previous experiences, triggering long forgotten feelings associated with those memories. That's because a particular aroma triggers areas of the brain that influence your emotions, memory, cardiovascular functioning, and hormonal balance. Your body thinks you are there!

In fact, memories associated with scent influence us more than most of us realize. Realtors know that the smell of baking cookies, heightened by the aroma of vanilla, can sell a house because it reminds potential buyers of being nurtured. In fact, realtors can forgo the cookies and simply scent the air with a vanilla fragrance.

The Sweet Smell of Success

International Flavors and Fragrances, Inc. (IFF), a New Jersey research company, has tested more than 2,000 people to better understand how certain scents summon deep-seated memories and affect personality, behavior, and sleep patterns. They found that pleasant smells put people into better moods and make them more willing to negotiate, cooperate, and compromise.

As a result of these and other studies, several large Tokyo corporations circulate the essential oils of lemon, peppermint, and cypress in their air-conditioning systems to keep workers alert and attentive on the job. As a happy side-effect, this practice is said to reduce the employees' urge to smoke. Pleasing fragrances are being pumped into offices, stores, and hotels in cities around the world to make the atmosphere more relaxing and invigorating, a task that multidimensional essential oils handle with ease. Of course, what these companies really want is for you to feel so comfortable that you will stay longer and return often.

Natural Uppers and Downers

Memory and association are only one way scents affect us psychologically. According to researchers studying aromacology, the science of medicinal aromas, fragrance actually alters our brain waves.

For instance, stimulating scents such as peppermint and eucalyptus intensify brain waves, making the mind sharper and clearer. The effects are similar to those of coffee, but are achieved without caffeine's detrimental impact on the adrenal glands. As a result, aroma is currently helping workers such as truck drivers and air traffic controllers, whose jobs—and the safety of others—depend on their being attentive.

Certain fragrances can also produce the opposite effect. If you inhale a flowery draft of chamomile tea, your brain waves will lengthen, causing you to feel relaxed. This is similar to the effect of taking a sedative drug but without the concomitant liver damage.

Some essential oils have effects similar to antidepressant drugs, according to the Olfaction Research Group at Warwick University in England. Italian psychiatrist Paolo Rovesti, M.D., helped is patients overcome depression using the scents of various citruses, such as orange, bergamot, lemon, and lemon verbena.

Psychologists help people overcome anxiety, tension, and mood swings by having them associate a scent with feelings of rest and contentment. The psychologist uses biofeedback or visualization techniques to help the client relax, and then sniff a relaxing scent. Later, the client can simply smell the relaxation scent when he or she becomes nervous or anxious.

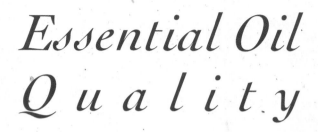

Essential Oil Quality

In order to be an educated consumer and purchase good quality essential oils for aromatherapy, you need to understand how an essential oil is extracted from the plant as well as what differentiates a good quality essential oil from a poor quality one. You can't tell just by looking. But using a high quality oil is essential to achieving maximum healing benefits from your aromatherapy treatments. And, in the long run, buying high quality oils will be easier on your pocketbook, too.

How Essential Oils Are Produced

There are several different ways to extract essential oils, and all require elaborate equipment. As you will see from the following descriptions, most extraction techniques are based on the fact that the majority of essential oils mix with oils, fats, alcohol, and certain solvents, but not with water. Some methods are more suitable for certain plants than others, depending on the plant's chemical make-up.

Distillation

Most pure essential oils are extracted from plants through steam distillation. Freshly picked plants are suspended over boiling water, and the steam pulls the oils out of the plant. The steam rises, is captured in a vessel, and is pushed along tubing. Then the steam is rapidly cooled, causing it to condense back into water. Since water and essential oils do not mix, the two separate, and the essential oil is collected.

A byproduct of this distillation is the remaining water. Some plants contain aromatic compounds that are so water soluble, they remain in the water that is left over after distillation. Such waters are very fragrant and are prized by aromatherapists, who refer to them as hydrosols. In aromatherapy, hydrosols are used mostly in cosmetics to moisturize skin.

Expression

The most direct method of producing essential oils is pressing them from the plant's flesh, seeds, and skins—a process similar to that used to obtain olive oil. This technique is used mostly with citrus peels, such as orange, lemon, lime, or grapefruit, because the oil in their peels is easily pressed out.

Enfleurage

This very old method is rarely used today except in France. It is a long and complicated process that has become very expensive. Blossoms are set on sheets of warm fat that absorb

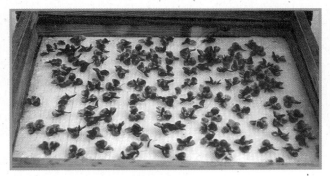

Violet petals release their essential oils into warm fat.

the oil from the flowers. Originally animal fat or lard was used, but now vegetable fats are more common. Once the essential oil has been incorporated into the fat, the "exhausted" flowers are removed and replaced with fresh ones. The process is repeated several times until the fat is infused with fragrance. Then the fat is separated out with solvents, leaving just the essential oil.

Solvents

Aromatherapists tend to shy away from oils obtained through chemical solvents, worrying that slight traces of the solvent may remain even though they are supposed to be completely removed. First, the plant is dissolved in a solvent such as benzene, hexane, or chlorure of methylene. The solvent, which has a low boiling point, is then evaporated off, sometimes with the help of a machine that uses vacuum or centrifugal force to help pull it away from the essential oil. The resulting oils are called "absolutes." A similar method uses paraffin waxes as the solvent, but does not evaporate them off. Instead, the remaining paraffins cause the final product to be solid, and thus it is called "concrete."

Even though the evaporated solvent is recaptured and cooled back into liquid so that it can be reused, this process is still expensive. As a result, it is reserved for costly oils that cannot be distilled, such as jasmine and vanilla, or for rose essential oil, which is slightly less expensive when obtained through this process rather than through distillation.

Carbon Dioxide

New methods of obtaining essential oils are currently being introduced. One of the most interesting processes, although extremely expensive, extracts the oil with carbon dioxide. The delightful result is an essential oil scent that is very close to that of the plant itself.

Quality

Since they are products of nature, the quality of essential oils is affected by growing conditions, the particular species of plant, extraction techniques, and storage, among other factors. Even the type of soil, temperature, and cloud cover affect some oils.

To determine the quality of an essential oil, you'll need to be concerned with three crucial characteristics—purity, grade, and integrity. The information below and lots of experience will guide you.

Purity

Purity is an important concern to anyone purchasing essential oils. They can be adulterated, cut, or entirely replaced with a cheaper substitute or extended or diluted with vegetable oils, alcohol, or solvents. These substitutes and extenders might not be derived from a plant at all.

But even if they are (see "Integrity," page 52), the oil will not be as potent as it should be, nor will it function as expected. Unfortunately, a label claiming a product is a pure essential oil is no guarantee that it is the real thing. An oil labelled rose or vanilla may have been produced in a laboratory out of synthetic chemicals, but it can still be labeled an essential oil.

Inexpensive oils such as orange, cedar, or peppermint are seldom altered. However, alteration is common with expensive oils that are in great demand, such as rose, melissa, and jasmine.

Dilution with vegetable oil is usually easy to detect (see page 55). Dilution with alcohol may be a bit more difficult to determine, but these oils do have a slight alcohol odor. Oils adulterated with a clear, non-oily solvent are the most difficult to recognize. This is a potential health hazard as well, since such solvents are readily absorbed into the body when rubbed on the skin or inhaled through the lungs.

Grades

Many essential oils are sold to distributors in different grades. Their prices often reflect this: The better grades command up to double the cost of the lesser grades. For example, lavender is commonly available in at least a dozen different grades and lemon in four. The lesser grades are often still pure essential oil, but they contain less of the most important aromatic principles.

Different processing methods can produce different grades. For example, redistillation produces oil that is stronger in some compounds than others. This is typically done with peppermint oil so the chewing gum and candy it flavors has a lighter, fresher taste and smell.

Once your nose has had a little experience with essential oils, you'll find that higher grades generally are more intense and carry a richer bouquet of fragrance. Lower quality oils usually smell less complicated or weak because they do not contain a full range of aromatic compounds.

When two bottles of the same kind of oil smell differently, it does not necessarily mean that one is better than the other. The best quality oils are similar to fine wine in that even experts don't agree on their favorites. For example, one geranium essential oil might carry a distinctly stronger hint of citrus while another smells more like rose. Which is better? Most people will prefer the rose, but that doesn't make it better.

Integrity

By integrity we mean that the oil is pure and natural and comes from a single species of plant (and probably even from the same region and harvest). An oil with integrity is not whipped up in a laboratory or composed of cheaper essential oils. But inexpensive lemongrass or citronella essential oils sometimes masquerade as the very expensive melissa (lemon balm) oil. To make an artificial rose oil in the laboratory, rose geranium may be used as a starting point, then chemically altered to mimic, although never completely accurately, a rose scent.

The problem here is that although the end product still contains only pure, natural essential oils, it will not have the properties you want and expect. Asking for an oil by its Latin name may help, but it doesn't guarantee that you will get what you want.

Shopping for Essential Oils

At first, it may seem a formidable task to detect the difference between good and poor grades of oil or to spot a synthetic. But you'll be pleasantly surprised at how easy it becomes, after only a little practice, to sniff out good essential oils.

Until your nose knows, you'll have to trust your source. Each essential oil company decides the quality it will offer. Some companies consistently sell the poorer, cheaper grades while others prefer to sell the higher grades. They will rarely offer you, as a retail consumer, a choice in grades. As a result, some lines tend to be more expensive than others. But do not use price alone to judge an oil's quality, since lower grades of oil may be sold for far more than they are worth. Remember, too, that store clerks do not always know much about aromatherapy and may naively think that anything labeled an essential oil comes from the plant named.

Sophisticated advertising and fancy packaging may also be misleading. And, because not everyone cares about the healing effects, a few companies have filled the growing demand for scents with the cheapest means at their disposal. The most unscrupulous will sell low quality oils for the price of better ones.

This being said, you will find oils and related supplies at natural food stores, herb stores, specialty mail-order catalogs, and of course, at aromatherapy and skin care outlets. Some stores also have retail sites on the Internet. (See the resource chapter for sources.)

Some essential oil mail-order companies are run by aromatherapists who stake their reputation on supplying high quality oils, so they may be the best way for you to get what you want. However, you need to know exactly what you want since you will not have the opportunity to sniff before purchase.

Price

There is great variation in the price of essential oils because some are more expensive to produce. In Bulgaria, schoolgirls labor in the misty morning, picking delicate rose petals just before the hot rays of the sun can release the fragrant oils into the air. Bulgaria produces the world's

TRICKS OF THE TRADE FOR BUYING ESSENTIAL OILS

Shopping for essential oils can be confusing. How can you, as a consumer, make educated decisions on what to buy? A few tricks of the trade should help you sniff your way through all the confusion.

• Buy from companies that have established a reputation for quality.

• When buying from an unknown company, purchase only one or two of their oils in small amounts (a quarter ounce, dram, or even less), even though it will cost proportionately more than a larger quantity.

• Put one drop of the essential oil on a piece of paper. Most oils are so volatile they will evaporate quickly, leaving no oily mark. The presence of an oil mark indicates that it's been adulterated. A few highly pigmented oils such as the deep blue German chamomile or brown patchouli will leave color stains, but they will not look or feel oily.

• If you are lucky enough to sniff and compare many oils, you will quickly develop a scent overload. Breathe several times through a scarf or cap of pure wool to clear your smell receptors.

• Check for scents that are fuller, rounder, and more complex. A little goes a long way, so you will need to use less in your products.

finest rose oil, but it takes about 600 pounds of petals to make a single ounce of oil! Rose oil also is expensive because the flowers must be carefully cultivated, pruned, and hand-picked.

Jasmine oil is expensive for similar reasons. Producing an ounce of pure jasmine requires 20 days labor for an experienced picker, followed by costly methods of extraction. As a result, rose and jasmine demand top dollar. On the other hand, peppermint is much less costly because the plant contains more essential oil, is relatively easy to grow and tend, and is harvested with machinery. The price of essential oils varies from $5 to an incredible $800 an ounce or more, reflecting the difficulty involved in their production.

Many other factors, such as difficult growing conditions, the rarity of the plant, or where the plant is grown, affect essential oil prices. Essential oils produced in the United States automatically demand a higher price to cover the greater costs of labor.

Surprisingly, cheaper oils will probably end up costing you more in the long run. Lesser quality oils are often weaker than high quality ones, and you will have to use more of them to achieve the same effect as a smaller amount of the high quality oil. Depending on how much more you have to use, you may end up spending more than if you'd simply purchased the better quality oil to begin with.

Storage

Once you've purchased quality essential oils, you certainly will want to keep them that way. Store them in glass containers. Some essential oils can actually dissolve plastic, and storing them even temporarily in it may contaminate the oil. Don't store essential oils in dropper bottles either, as it doesn't take long for the rubber seals and squeeze bulbs to melt into a gooey mess.

The color of the bottle doesn't really matter. Just be sure to keep all essential oils out of direct sunlight and away from heat so they don't lose their potency.

Essential oils are natural preservatives and will help preserve your carrier oils. Their scent will change and fade over time, however, and eventually lose its quality. Properly stored, most oils will keep for at least several years. The citrus oils, such as orange and lemon, are most vulnerable to losing their smell, but even they will keep for a couple of years if refrigerated.

A few essential oils, including patchouli, clary sage, benzoin, vetiver, and sandalwood, actually help fix the scent of other aromas combined with them. And they get better with age. The same is true for thick resins such as myrrh. Patchouli that has been stored for many years smells so rich, few people recognize it—even those who otherwise dislike it! Essential oils such as these become yet more valuable with age.

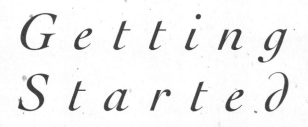

Getting
Started

Making aromatherapy products to use for healing or as skin care products is as easy as it is fun. And you don't need much in the way of equipment to get started. In fact, you probably have most of what you need in your kitchen already. Add some bottles, some essential oils, and some carrier oils to your supplies and, using the explanations and recipes in this book, you'll be ready to begin experimenting.

Supplies

A measuring cup, measuring spoons, and perhaps some small funnels will start you on the
road to aromatherapy production. Unless you
are adding essential oils to a ready-made product, you will need appropriate bottles or containers for storage. Simple bottles and vials are
sold at drugstores; for fancier ones, check out
your local natural food store. Mail order sources
(see the Resources chapter) offer a greater variety of containers. Buy some labels for the bottles, too. Make sure to have paper towels and
rubbing alcohol on hand for clean up.

You will need a way to measure small amounts
of the essential oils and transfer them from bottle to bottle. Some essential oils are sold in bottles that have an insert called a reducer that
allows only a drop of oil to come out at a time. It
may take a few tries to get comfortable using it,
but do not shake the bottle or several drops will
come out at once. Glass droppers work well for
obtaining just the right amount of essential oil
and are sold in drugstores, some natural food
stores, and by some essential oil suppliers.

Be careful not to contaminate your essential
oils by putting a dropper from one oil into another, but you don't need a separate dropper for
each oil. Simply rinse the dropper in rubbing alcohol and wait a few minutes for the alcohol to
completely evaporate before putting it into an-

other oil. Having two or three droppers allows you to rotate them for rinsing and drying.

If you prefer, use a long, narrow tube called a pipette to measure out small amounts of essential oils. Pipettes can be made of glass or plastic; however, the easiest to use — but hardest to clean — is plastic with a squeeze bulb at one end. Practice with these using water before attempting to get exact measurements with your essential oils. Pipettes are sold in chemical equipment catalogs, some drugstores, and aromatherapy supply catalogs.

To measure larger quantities, use a Pyrex measuring cup with a pour spout. A set of measuring spoons is also useful for measuring more than a few drops of essential oil. (See the box on page 67.) In addition to the equipment, you'll also need some essential oils (see the box on page 61 for suggested starter oils) and various carriers such as vegetable oil, distilled water, rubbing alcohol, and vodka. You can buy or order fancier vegetable oils, such as almond, apricot, grape seed, and jojoba, at most natural food stores.

Carriers

Mixing your essential oil with a carrier oil is the most popular way of preparing aromatherapy products. It is also the easiest way to dilute essential oils in preparation for use. There are several choices of carriers; the most common are

Basic Essential Oil Starter Kit

LAVENDER—fights infection, inflammation, insomnia, pain, depression, anxiety; appropriate for all complexion and hair types

CHAMOMILE—aids digestion and promotes relaxation; treats allergies, menstrual cramps, depression, inflammation, anxiety, anger, rashes, and dry and problem skin, complexion, and hair

ROSEMARY—relieves pain, congestion, constipation and grief; stimulates circulation and memory; appropriate for most complexion and hair types

TEA TREE—fights most types of infection; appropriate for oily skin and hair

PEPPERMINT—relieves indigestion, sinus congestion, itching, and panic; mental stimulant; use small amounts for dry skin and hair

LEMON, ORANGE, OR OTHER CITRUS— antidepressant; kills parasites; appropriate for oily complexion and hair

GERANIUM—balances mind and body; appropriate for all complexion and hair types vegetable oil, alcohol, water, and more rarely, vinegar. The carrier you choose will depend on how you plan to apply your treatment. For a massage or body oil, vegetable oil is the best choice. For a liniment, you may prefer alcohol as your base because it doesn't leave an oily residue. A room spray only needs a water base, while aloe vera juice is perfect for a complexion spray. The recipes given in the Application Formulas chapter specify the best carrier for each situation.

You can also dilute essential oils in ready-made products that use vegetable oils as their base, such as salves, creams, or lotions that you purchase at the store. This is a quick way to custom-make your own products. Select products that have little or no essential oils in them already to ensure that you do not end up with too much scent in the finished product. Many natural food stores sell unscented cream, lotion, and shampoo bases.

Vegetable Oil

Essential oils blend well into vegetable oils. Vegetable oils have other advantages, too: They are soothing to the skin, hold moisture in, and are easy to apply. Any high-quality vegetable oil such as almond, apricot, hazelnut, olive, grape seed, or sesame can be a carrier oil. You don't necessarily need to use "cold-pressed" oil. In fact, you should avoid the heavily scented olive and peanut oils because they have their own odor, which will cover up the scent of the essential oils you are using.

Vegetable oil's molecules are too large to penetrate the skin as essential oil molecules do, but they slide smoothly over one another and over the skin, making them ideal for cosmetic products. Eventually, when you're more familiar with the properties of the various oils, you may vary the oil according to the application. But when starting out, use any of the carrier oils listed earlier. Store the carrier oils away from heat and light to ensure their freshness. Keep the more expensive oils in the refrigerator if you won't be using them immediately.

Vitamin E oil is an excellent antioxidant, and adding it to any aromatherapy blend will help extend the life of most vegetable oils. One or two capsules (200 to 400 IUs) per two-ounce bottle of carrier is enough. Just prick the end of the capsule with a pin and squeeze. To ensure freshness, make only enough of a blend to last for a couple months or keep it refrigerated. If you plan to keep a blend for a long time and are worried about rancidity, consider using jojoba oil. While more expensive than most, jojoba oil will never go rancid. If you're pinching pennies, use it as just a portion of your blend.

Alcohol

The same proportions suggested for diluting essential oils into vegetable oil will also work for alcohol. Although it is not used as often, alcohol is antiseptic and cooling and quickly evaporates, leaving no oily residue. You may choose between using a drinking alcohol, such as vodka, or a rubbing alcohol, which is poisonous. If you choose drinking alcohol, any type will work, but vodka is often used because it has no additional flavors or additives. An 80-proof vodka is 40 percent alcohol and 60 percent water. If you use rubbing alcohol (alcohol made from wood), be sure that it is not ingested. By itself, alcohol is far too drying to use on the skin or hair. Witch hazel, which is a blend of alcohol plus an extract of the bark and leaves of the *hamamelis virginiana*, makes a good base for a mild astringent.

Vinegar

A few aromatherapy preparations incorporate vinegar. It is actually a better base for both skin and hair than alcohol, but it is not as popular due to its strong smell. The smell dissipates rather quickly, however, and you'll be pleased with the result if you try it. Vinegar is antiseptic, although not as antiseptic as alcohol. Its acidity helps restore the acid mantle or pH-balance to the skin and hair. For this purpose, apple cider vinegar is best, although many people prefer white vinegar because it has no color. Vinegar is water soluble, so you can dilute it with distilled water if you find its smell or sting too strong for the product you are making. Distilled water is used because it doesn't contain chlorine or other city water additives and has none of the bacteria found in well water.

Water

For aromatherapy, you will primarily be adding a few drops of an essential oil blend to your bath, to a bowl of hot water for compresses, or to cold water in a bottle that you will spray. Nonchlorinated or distilled water is always preferred. Fill the containers with hot water before you add the essential oils so they won't evaporate too rapidly.

Dilutions

Some people find it easier to measure drops, others prefer measuring essential oils by the teaspoon. It depends on how much you need to measure at one time and the width of the container into which it's going. The size of a drop varies, depending on the size of the dropper opening and the temperature and viscosity (thickness) of the essential oil. Teaspoons are usually more convenient if you are preparing large quantities.

Most aromatherapy applications are a two-percent dilution. This means 2 drops of essential oil is added for every 100 drops of carrier oil—a safe and effective dilution for most aromatherapy applications. A one-percent dilution is suggested for children, pregnant women, and those who are weak from chronic illness. In some cases, you will want to use even less. Dilutions of three percent or more are used only for strong preparations such as liniments or for "spot" therapy, when you are only treating a tiny area instead of the entire body. Always remember that in aromatherapy, more is not necessarily better. In fact, too great a concentration may produce unwanted reactions. (Be sure to review the safety information on pages 91–92.) The following are standard dilutions:

- 1 percent dilution: 5–6 drops per ounce of carrier
- 2 percent dilution: 10–12 drops (about ⅛ teaspoon) per ounce of carrier
- 3 percent dilution: 15–18 drops (a little less than ¼ teaspoon) per ounce of carrier

Blending

For your very first aromatherapy blends, keep it simple. Use your favorite essential oils, but preferably no more than three to five at a time. Later, the many choices of oils will add to the excitement of creating your own blends.

Keep an aromatherapy notebook from the very beginning—you'll need exact records of how you made all your preparations. Jot down the ingredients, proportions, and processing procedures you used for each blend, as well as observations about how well it worked. Label

Measurement Conversions

12.5 drops = ⅛ teaspoon = ¹⁄₄₈ oz = ⅙ dram =
about ⅝ ml.

25 drops = ¼ teaspoon = ¹⁄₂₄ oz = ⅓ dram =
about 1¼ ml.

75 drops = ¾ teaspoon = ⅛ oz = 1 dram =
about 3.7 ml.

100 drops = 1 teaspoon = ⅙ oz = 1⅓ dram =
about 5 ml.

your finished products with the ingredients, date, and special instructions, if any. You will be thankful for this information later when you come up with a formula everyone loves, and you want to duplicate it.

When considering blends, try to think about the characteristics of each oil, including what professional perfumers call *personality, aroma notes,* and *odor intensity.* Perfumers think of each oil as having its own unique personality, and they think of scent in terms of a musical scale: Fragrances have head or top notes, middle or heart notes, and base notes. The top notes are the odors that are smelled first but evaporate quickly, the heart is the scent that emerges after the first fifteen minutes, while the base note is the scent that lingers hours later.

Essential oils vary in odor intensity, which may or may not correspond to the evaporation rate of the aroma notes. Add much smaller amounts of strong essential oils, as it is extremely easy for an especially potent oil such as rosemary to completely overpower the soft scent of an oil such as sandalwood or cedar. When mixing small experimental quantities, one drop of a high intensity oil such as cinnamon can be way too much. Try adding just a smidgen of oil with the end of a toothpick. You can tell which oils have a high odor intensity, such as patchouli and cinnamon, just by smelling them. Use only about one drop of any of these oils to five drops of a more subtle essential oil, such as lavender. On the other hand, orange has such a low odor intensity, you will need about eight drops of it to blend evenly with four drops of lavender.

Here you have the makings of a formula: 8 drops orange, 4 drops lavender, and 1 drop clary sage. This formula presents a lesson in intensity and is arranged by notes. The scent leans toward the top and middle note regions. The orange brightens the top, evaporating relatively quickly, while the clary sage provides a sweetly sauntering base for comforting lavender.

There are many ways to alter the formula. For instance, add a drop of cinnamon instead of the clary sage for a scent that's a little more spicy and stimulating. If you want the woodsy smell of cedar, add several drops to balance the blend. The options are almost endless.

Another way to expand a blend is to choose oils that have similar characteristics. It will make your blend seem more complicated and mysterious because no one can pinpoint exactly what the aroma is. Try combining peppermint and spearmint, lemon and bergamot, or cinnamon and ginger. Using oils that come from different parts of a plant tends to deepen and enrich the scent. For instance, add just the tiniest amount of turpentinelike juniper needles to a rich juniper berry to create a more detailed fullness.

Incorporating Herbs

Herbs can be important and effective adjuncts to aromatherapy treatments. In fact, herbs and essential oils used together provide greater healing benefits than does either one alone. The herbs will lend their own less concentrated but more complete medicinal properties.

Oils made by macerating (soaking) herbs in vegetable oils are called infused oils. These can replace plain vegetable oils in aromatherapy preparations to make a more potent medicine. You can buy an infused oil or make your own.

Buying an herbal salve, lotion, or cream and stirring essential oils into it is a quick way to make an herb and essential oil combination. Try to find herbal products that contain little or no essential oil, because you don't want to end up with too much essential oil in the final product.

Application Formulas

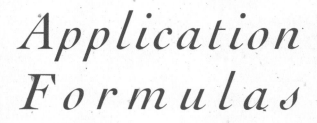

Making your own aromatherapy products has many advantages. You can be certain that your homemade products contain only the highest quality ingredients, yet they will likely cost only a fraction of what you'd pay for them in the store. And you'll get the satisfaction of making delightful preparations to give as gifts to family and friends — not to mention yourself!

Using essential oils — rather than the whole herb — will eliminate complex procedures. Your finished product can usually be ready in a few minutes instead of hours.

Medicinal Preparations

In this section you will find a general overview and explanation of essential oil application techniques. This will help you determine what type of product you need to buy or make to best suit your needs. You will find essential oil recipes for specific ailments and beauty care, utilizing the following preparation techniques, in the Common Ailments chapter. Keep a few essential oils on hand, such as those in the essential oil starter kit (see page 61), so you'll be prepared to treat everyday problems. Just be sure to store them out of the reach of children.

Compress

An aromatherapy compress concentrates essential oils in a specific area of the body and keeps the area moist. It is one of the quickest and easiest therapeutic techniques to make. Add about 5 drops of an essential oil or a blend of oils to a cup of water. Use hot or cold water, whichever is best for the particular treatment: Cold water helps relieve itching, swelling, and inflammation, while hot water increases circulation and opens pores, helping to flush out blemishes. Fold a soft cloth and soak it in the water; then wring it out and apply it where needed. If you feel overheated, try a cold compress on your forehead. Cold is also usually the preferred temperature for relieving strained eyes. A cool compress can also help to get rid of a headache, although a few people find that heat works better for them. A hot compress against the back of the neck will relieve neck strain and tight muscles.

Foot or Hand Bath

Soaking your hands or feet in an aromatherapy mini-bath is an excellent treatment for stiffness, aches, and skin irritations. In fact, your entire body will benefit since the essential oils penetrate the skin and enter the bloodstream. To make a foot or hand bath, simply add 5 to 10 drops of essential oil to a quart of hot or cold water in a large basin. Stir well to distribute the essential oils, then soak your feet or hands for at least five minutes. Cold water reduces swelling while warm water relaxes stiff muscles. To improve leg circulation in conditions such as varicose veins, alternate between a hot and cold bath.

Gargle, Mouthwash, or Throat Spray

A spray or gargle brings essential oils into direct contact with the bacteria or virus responsible for causing sore throat or laryngitis. To make either one, dissolve ½ teaspoon salt in about ¼ cup water and add 1–2 drops of an antiseptic essential oil such as tea tree. Shake or stir well. Be sure to spit out the gargle or mouthwash — essential oils should not be swallowed.

Inhalant

Steam inhalations are a great way to treat any upper respiratory or sinus problem. The steam carries essential oils directly to sinuses and lungs, where they fight infection. Additionally, the warm, moist air opens nasal and bronchial passages, making it easier to breathe. To create a steam inhalant, bring about 3 cups of water to a boil in a pan. Turn off the heat, and add 3–5 drops of essential oil to the water. Drape a towel over both your head and the pan to capture the steam, keeping your eyes closed and your head about 12 inches from the water. Take deep, relaxing breaths of the fragrant steam. You can also humidify and disinfect an entire room — just keep the mixture on a very low simmer. Essential oils can also be used in many humidifiers.

When you're away from home and steam inhalation treatments are impractical, inhale a tissue scented with the oils or use a natural nasal inhaler, which can be found at natural food stores.

Liniment

Liniments increase circulation. Rub them externally on the skin to warm muscles and to reduce muscle and joint pain. Liniments also dis-infect wounds and dry up skin eruptions. Fitness experts suggest applying liniment before exercising, not afterwards, so that it can work like a mini-warm-up, heating muscles so they will stretch better. (Don't use this as an excuse to skimp on your stretches, however!) Make a quick and easy liniment by adding 15–20 drops of the appropriate heating essential oils, such as cinnamon, peppermint, and clove, for every ounce of alcohol, oil, or vinegar. Alcohol is cooling and quickly evaporates, leaving no oily residue. Oil heats up faster and stays on the skin longer, making it more like a concentrated massage.

Massage/Body Oil

Massage oil consists of essential oils blended in a carrier oil (see pages 60 and 62 for a discussion of carrier oils). A small amount of healing essential oil can thus be evenly distributed over a large area of the body. Rubbing warms the body, relaxes muscles, relieves stress, encourages deep breathing, and helps the oils to penetrate deeply. All of these do their part in treating the whole person, rather than just focusing on a single symptom. To make either a massage or body oil, combine ½ teaspoon (50 drops) of essential oil with 4 ounces of any vegetable oil. A body oil made from essential oils is also a good alternative when the patient won't swallow a pill or drink tea. For example, if a child with a stomachache refuses to take any medicine, rub a therapeutic body oil on his or her stomach.

Salve

Salves are made of herbal oils that are thickened with beeswax, so they form a healing and protective coating that adheres better to the skin. They are used on almost all skin problems, such as minor cuts, bruises, scrapes, diaper or heat rash, insect bites, eczema, psoriasis, and swelling. You can make any salve aromatherapeutic by stirring 24 drops of essential oil into 2 ounces of salve. This is fairly easy to do with a toothpick. The resulting salve will be a little runnier than usual, but it will stick to the skin perfectly well.

Sitz Bath

A "sitz" bath is simply a mini-bath that employs hot and cold water to increase blood circulation, primarily in the pelvic region. This makes it ideal for uterine or bladder problems. Add 5–10 drops of essential oil to a bathtub containing about 10 inches of water (up to your waist). The water temperature should be as hot as you can easily stand but not so hot as to hurt. Prepare a small tub of cold water and leave it nearby. Sit in the hot water 5 to 10 minutes. Quickly remove yourself to the tub of cold water and sit in it for at least 1 minute. The large plastic tubs sold at hardware stores are well-suited for this purpose. Continue alternating between the hot and cold tubs for a total of two to five times each. Repeat the treatment every day for 3 to 5 days. Unless otherwise stated in the Common Ailments chapter, rosemary is a good general oil for this purpose.

Cosmetic Preparations

Pamper yourself with the luxurious feeling of aromatherapy skin care facials. Once you've discovered how beautiful they make you feel, you might want to make it a weekly treat. And you even may want to invite your friends over for an afternoon of preparing and applying a whole skin care regime. Your afternoon could begin with a mask of cosmetic clay. While waiting for the clay to dry, you can massage each other's feet using scented massage oil. When the clay is dry, rinse it off with warm water and follow with an oatmeal scrub. Then enjoy a relaxing facial steam. Spray your face with a fine aromatic water, and while your skin is still moist, apply a soothing cream or lotion. Finish with a drop of essential oil perfume. Preparation formulas for these skin care processes and others follow.

Aromatic Waters

Scented waters treat many different skin problems, such as acne and burns, and are also used cosmetically as a skin-freshener. The essential oils they contain are so diluted that aromatic waters can be applied directly onto sensitive areas of the face. They are perfect for making herbal compresses for injured skin or for complexion problems. Although different from hydrosols, which are the more expensive by-products of distilling essential oils (see Healing Benefits chapter), these aromatic waters work wonderfully in their own right. Add 5–10 drops of fragrant essential oils to 4 ounces of water or aloe vera juice.

Aromatic Bath

Bathing offers the most relaxing and luxurious way to take your medicine! Since stress makes

FLOATING AROMATIC BATH OIL

½ teaspoon essential oil (your choice)
1 ounce vegetable oil

Combine ingredients. Use 1 teaspoon per bath. For babies, use only 1 drop in a basin. This is especially good for dry skin. When you emerge, your body is covered with a light film of fragrant oil that lasts for hours. It also keeps your skin from becoming dry or itchy after bathing.

you more susceptible to disease, an herbal bath may be the most important herbal treatment we have. Not only is the bath relaxing, it allows the medicinal essential oils to be absorbed gently over a large area of the body. Baths are also useful in treating certain skin problems and muscle pains. The essential oil-laden steam that rises off an aromatherapy bath can double as an inhalant for lung and sinus congestion.

The easiest way to create an aromatherapy bath is to add 3 to 5 drops of essential oils di-

BATH SALTS

½ teaspoon essential oil (your choice)
1 cup borax
½ cup sea salt
½ cup baking soda

Mix salts together, and add essential oils, mixing well to combine. Use ¼ to ½ cup of the bath salts per bath. For muscle aches and pains, add ½ cup Epsom salts to this recipe. (All of these salts are sold in grocery stores.) This makes a very relaxing and soothing bath. Sea salt softens water and makes more soap suds, so you can use much less soap. This is good because soap can be harsh on delicate skin. This mix also makes the skin feel smooth, although in excess, it may be drying to already dry skin.

rectly to your bath water. Add them after you run the water so they won't evaporate too quickly, and be sure to swirl the oils around before you get in. Avoid using more than one drop of hot oils such as peppermint, and go easy on the citrus oils, especially orange, for the same reason. Want to make your bathing experience even more deluxe? Then try the aromatherapy recipes on pages 77 and 78.

Cosmetic Clay

Bentonite or cosmetic clay, which are available at natural food stores in boxes and in bulk, can be used as a facial mask for tightening the skin. To prepare, add 1 to 2 teaspoons of distilled water to 1 tablespoon of clay to make it into a paste. (Usually one part water to two parts clay will do.) Add 3 drops of essential oil and stir in well. Pat over your face, let dry, and then wash off with warm water. Clay can also be used medicinally for drawing out bee stings or for drying rashes and pimples.

Cream

You can turn any basic cream or lotion into an aromatherapeutic product. Start with an unscented cream, and stir in 3–6 drops essential oil for every ounce of cream or lotion—or make your own cream from scratch using the recipe on page 80.

CREAM

1 cup oil
¾ ounce beeswax (22 grams), shaved
1 cup distilled water, warm
30 to 50 drops essential oils

Making cream is very similar to making mayonnaise—the proportions need to be fairly exact for it to come out right. Carefully melt the shaved beeswax in the oil on the stove. Cool it so that you can put your finger in a oil without discomfort. Put the lid on your blender with the center cap removed. Pour the warm water into the blender through a funnel (using a wide mouth funnel reduces splattering). Turn the blender on high speed, and add the oil/beeswax mixture slowly and evenly. It should begin to thicken after about three fourths of the oil has been added. This is a good time to add the essential oils. When all of the oil has been added, you will have a thick, beautiful cream. Pour the cream into wide-mouth jars. The cream will last at least a month if kept in a cool place. Storing it in the refrigerator will prolong its shelf life for several months.

Lotion

Making lotion is a little trickier than cream, but it can certainly be done in your kitchen. Use the following ingredients, and follow instructions given for making cream (opposite).

LOTION

¾ cup oil
½ ounce beeswax, shaved (about 2 tablespoons)
1 cup distilled water, warm
30 drops essential oils

- Do not cut these recipes or there will not be enough liquid to cover the blender's blades.

- To vary the recipe, the water portion of your cream can be any one, or a combination, of water-soluble ingredients such as aloe vera juice, rose water, or a strong herbal tea.

Underarm Deodorant

The most important action of any deodorant is to kill bacteria, which essential oils do very well. By making your own deodorant, you can soothe rash and irritation (try Roman chamomile) and avoid the use of harsh, pore-blocking ingredients found in commercial products.

DEODORANT

15 drops lavender
5 drops sage oil
5 drops coriander
2 ounces aloe vera juice or witch hazel

Combine all ingredients in a spray bottle.
Shake well before each use.
This will keep at least a year.

Perfume

Commercial perfumes only imitate the glory of nature. Why not wear a bit of nature itself as your personal fragrance? Apply one undiluted drop of nonirritating essential oil to a spot where your pulse beats, such as your inner wrist or behind the ear, and the warmth generated will help spread the scent. You might want to start with floral oils, such as lavender or geranium, or one of the aromatic woods, such as sandalwood. Some people prefer the wild scent of patchouli. Others splurge on the more pricey rose, jasmine, or neroli (orange blossom), all of which are found in expensive perfumes.

Lip Balm

Protect your lips from drying wind and cold conditions by using soothing lip balm. Heal chapped lips and keep them kissable while enjoying natural flavors such as tangerine, lemon, peppermint, rose, or even anise, by using the following recipe:

LIP BALM

¼ cup of your favorite oil
¼ ounce beeswax, shaved
10 drops essential oil

Warm the oil in a pan and add the beeswax. Stir until the wax melts. Add essential oils after the salve cools just a bit so the oils do not evaporate. Store the balm in a snap top "lip balm" container, which are sold in drugstores and camping supply shops. They may also be available at your natural food store. Lip balm will last at least a year unless you keep it in a warm place such as your car.

Facial Steam

A facial steam will open the pores of your face, making your skin feel dewy soft as it takes on a radiant, youthful pink glow. Bring one quart of water to a simmer, remove from heat, and add 15 drops of essential oils. (Try five drops each of lavender, rosemary, and geranium.) Keeping your head about 12 inches above the pan, place a towel over the back of your head and secure the ends around the pan to capture the steam in a miniature sauna. Be sure to keep your eyes closed so they won't become irritated. Steam for a few minutes, then lift your head and take a breath of fresh air as needed. Go back under the towel and repeat a few times. Do this for no longer than five or ten minutes — less if you have sensitive skin.

Skin Scrub

Grind 3 tablespoons of oatmeal with 1 table-spoon cornmeal in an electric coffee grinder. Store powder in a closed container. To use the scrub, moisten 1 teaspoon with enough aromatic water (see above), tea, or hydrosol to make a paste. Apply to dampened face. Gently scrub and rinse with warm water.

Preparations for Around the Home

Diffuser

The most refined, but expensive, way to scent a room is with an aromatic diffuser. Diffusers are small electrical units that pump unheated fragrance into the room. Unheated scent is more pure than heated scent. There is quite a variety of diffusers available; they cost from approximately $60 to $120, depending upon capacity and style. Directions will come with the diffuser when you buy it. Generally, you place a few drops of essential oil in a hand-blown glass container and turn on a small compressor that's connected with a piece of tubing. The glass unit disperses a fine mist of microparticles mixed with the stream of air produced by the pump. By increasing the surface area of the scent molecules, it becomes extremely effective at disinfecting and energizing the atmosphere. Another advantage to the diffuser is that the vapor of essential oil can be directed into the nose or throat. It can also be used in a sick room for 10 to 15 minutes every hour to clear airborne bacteria that may spread infection.

Do not use thick oils such as vetiver, sandalwood, vanilla, myrrh, or benzoin in the diffuser, as they don't evaporate easily. However, these oils can be diluted with thinner oils such as the citruses, eucalyptus, and rosemary or mixed with alcohol. Don't let a diffuser sit with essential oil in it without occasionally turning it on because the oils will eventually oxidize and thicken. Sometimes expressed citrus oils contain a bit of sediment that may clog your diffuser. To clean or unclog it, soak the glass unit in alcohol, and depending on the model, unplug the opening with a pin or toothpick. Then rinse the unit, and let it air dry.

Light Bulb Ring

Ceramic or metal rings designed to be placed directly on light bulbs are available at many stores. Place 2–3 drops on the ring while it's cold, and be sure not to touch it again until it cools down after turning off the light. You can also place a couple drops of essential oil directly on the bulb, although the oil doesn't last as long.

Potpourri

Few things grace a room more than an attractive container of dried flowers, herbs, woods, and spices, freshening a room with its gentle and perhaps seasonal background aroma. Modern potpourris owe most of their fragrance to essential oils added to dried herbs. The basic recipe is ½ teaspoon essential oil to 2 cups dried herbs.

Since some essential oils have the unique property of becoming better with age, these can be used as fixatives. They will preserve the fragrance, making it last long after it would otherwise dissipate. The potpourri also smells better with the addition of such oils as patchouli, sandalwood, benzoin, clary sage, balsam of Peru, balsam of tolu, vetiver, and orris root, used either as the chopped herb or in the form of an essential oil. The most popular potpourri fixative is orris root. It has a light, violetlike fragrance that blends with any scent, and it is not over-powering. Although a few people are allergic to orris, it is still the all-time favorite. Its essential oil is so rare that orris is added in its chopped form.

POTPOURRI BASE

1 cup mixed herbs, dried
1 tablespoon orris root, chopped
¼ teaspoon essential oil
(twice the amount for simmering potpourri)

Use any combination of attractive flowers, leaves, bark, wood shavings, or cones for the dried plant material. Add the orris root and essential oils and stir. Keep the mixture in a closed container for several days so the scent can be absorbed by the plant material. This potpourri will stay fragrant for many months. When it gets faint, revive it with a few more drops of essential oil.

Potpourri Cooker

Simmering potpourri cookers have basins containing water and a potpourri mix which are suspended over and heated by a candle or electricity. When the water heats up, it releases the essential oil molecules into the air. Since only a small amount of potpourri is used, at least two or even three times the amount of essential oil is required.

Although you'll find potpourri mixes for all rooms and all seasons, you don't even need the potpourri. You can simply put a few drops of essential oil in water in the basin. When the water heats up, the molecules of essential oils float into the air.

Room Spray

Instantly change the energy in a room, cleanse the air, or get rid of unpleasant odors by using an aromatherapeutic room spray. The formula below is a multipurpose room disinfectant. It can be sprayed in a sick room or used on the kitchen

DISINFECTANT ROOM SPRAY

4 drops eucalyptus (or tea tree)
3 drops lavender
2 drops bergamot
2 drops thyme
1 drop peppermint
2 ounces water

Add the essential oils to the water. Keep in a spritzer bottle (sold in most drug stores and some cosmetic stores). Be sure to shake the bottle very well right before using to help distribute the essential oils in the water. Otherwise, they tend to float on the surface.

counter. You can also change the oils to create a spray that will make the room fragrant or that will impact the emotions. One mom, for instance, sprays her children's bedrooms every evening with a soothing chamomile and ylang ylang mix that helps relax them for sleep.

Sachet

Sachets freshen clothing and keep moths and other insects away.

MOTH-PROOF SACHET

20 drops cedarwood
8 drops lavender
8 drops patchouli or sage
1 dozen cotton balls

Combine essential oils and place about 3 drops on each cotton ball. Store in a closed container for a couple days. Place with clothes, using them instead of commercial moth balls (about six for an average sized box or suitcase). To make more attractive balls, tie a small fabric square around the cotton ball.

Scented Candle

Impregnated with essential oils, candles release the scent as they burn, creating whatever mood you want. You can make an aromatherapy candle from a purchased unscented candle by adding several drops of essential oil to the candle's wick. Wait 24 hours, until the wick absorbs the oil, before using the candle. You can make scented candles from scratch by adding oil to the melted wax or by saturating the wick just before pouring the candle. The wick method uses less oil, but many people like the scent of the candle.

CITRONELLA CANDLE

1 votive candle
20 drops citronella

Using a glass dropper, drop the oil on the candle's wick. Wait 24 hours before using. This particular candle is especially good for repelling bugs.

Vacuum Cleaner

Drop 2 to 4 drops of essential oil directly into the bag. Not only does the oil disinfect the dirt, but it will brighten your day. Try lemon eucalyptus—it is highly antiseptic, and the lemon gives people a feeling of cleanliness. In addition, its stimulating properties will help you get that housework done.

Washing Machine/Dryer

Put 1 or 2 drops on a cloth tossed into the dryer. Or add a few drops of citrus or lavender directly in the wash water to both scent and disinfect clothes. Of course, most laundry detergents are already heavily scented, so you don't want to overdo it.

Safety

Essential oils are potent substances that can be harmful if mishandled. Unlike an herb tea or tincture that is made with the whole herb, essential oils are extremely concentrated.

Work with essential oils in a well-ventilated space, and take frequent breaks while handling them. Overexposure to an oil either through the skin or by smelling can result in nausea, headache, skin irritation, emotional unease, or a "spaced out" feeling. If you find yourself feeling like this, get some fresh air right away. If you experience skin irritation, quickly dilute the oil by applying straight vegetable oil to the affected area. Water won't be as effective since essential oils are not soluble in water.

Don't apply essential oils directly on the skin, referred to in aromatherapy as "neat," because of the danger of overdose. The gentler oils, such as lavender, may occasionally be used undiluted on a very small area, say an insect bite or skin eruption. But rubbing just a few drops of most essential oils directly onto the skin could easily amount to ingesting the equivalent of 10 cups of herb tea all at once! In addition to irritating or even burning your skin, you could damage your liver and kidneys, which must detoxify large amounts of essential oils once they enter the blood stream. Damage to the liver or kidneys is not always readily apparent, so you could be injuring your health without even knowing it.

Be especially careful when using essential oils known to be skin irritants (allspice, bay, cinnamon, clove, oregano, sage, savory, thyme [except linalol], thuja, and wintergreen). Never use these with children, the elderly, people who are very ill with a chronic disease, or anyone with liver or kidney damage, asthma, or a heart problem. Instead, turn to less harmful alternatives. A good example is thyme oil. Even diluted applications can burn the skin, so substitute lemon thyme, which is much milder. Oregano essential oil is so potent that many aromatherapists will not use it. Instead, they use the closely related marjoram or lavender, which are equal if not better muscle relaxants and antiseptics.

Essential Oils

Essential oils, the fragrant, concentrated liquids extracted from the flowers, leaves, roots, bark, and fruit of an aromatic plant, are the main ingredients in aromatherapy treatments. Each oil has a unique scent as well as constituents that can treat many different conditions. The essential oils profiled in this chapter are among the most common, commercially available oils, and they are very versatile. The profiles will tell you about each oil's therapeutic and cosmetic uses, scent, and principal constituents. You'll also find some intriguing myths and folklore associated with the oils.

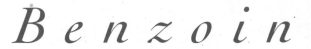

Benzoin

(Styrax benzoin)

Family: Styracaceae

It is the trunk of the tall Southeast Asian benzoin tree that, when cut, exudes a delicious, vanilla-scented gum resin. Used since antiquity in medicine and incense, the resin was imported by the Arabs to use as a less expensive substitute for frankincense. They made solid pomades that smelled like vanilla and were rubbed on the skin for both fragrance and healing. Arabian traders brought benzoin to Greece, Rome, and Egypt, where it became prized as a fixative in perfumes and potpourris—still one of its uses today. The Crusaders carried benzoin into Europe to scent their cherished Oriental-style perfume. Europeans highly regarded benzoin for its medicinal properties as well as its scent.

Benzoin is typically sold as an absolute, but it is so thick it may be difficult for you to get it out of the bottle. If so, dilute it with a little alcohol, such as vodka, or dissolve it in warm vegetable oil so it is easier to pour. An absolute thinned with ethyl glycol is also sold, but aromatherapists avoid oils and scents containing this chemical. You can also buy benzoin tincture in an alcohol base in drugstores.

PRINCIPAL CONSTITUENTS: Resin, benzoic acid, vanillin, coniferyl benzoate, phenylethylene, and phenylpropylic alcohol. Cinnamic acid occurs only in the type called Sumatra benzoin.

SCENT: It has a sweet, warm, vanillalike odor that is long lasting and makes it an excellent fixative.

THERAPEUTIC PROPERTIES: Antibacterial, antifungal; seals wounds from infection; counteracts inflammation; decreases gas, indigestion, and lung congestion; promotes circulation; and is an antioxidant and deodorant

USED FOR: Effective against redness, irritation, or itching on the skin, benzoin's most popular use is in a cream to protect chapped skin and improve skin elasticity. Since it is also a strong preservative, adding it to vegetable oil–based preparations delays their oxidation and spoilage. Benzoin essential oil can be added to chest rub balms and massage oils for lung and sinus ailments (stir in about 12 drops of essential oil per ounce of preparation), or use the tincture of benzoin to make cough medicine formulas.

Bergamot

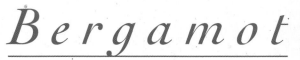

(Citrus bergamia)
Family: *Rutaceae*

Have you ever enjoyed a cup of Earl Grey tea? What makes this tea unique is the addition of bergamot essential oil, which flavors many beverages and candies. Bergamot's deep citrusy fragrance is also a popular component of men's fragrances.

A small citrus tree originally from tropical Asia, it produces the round, green fruit whose oils are expressed from the rinds before ripening. While not edible or pretty, they smell truly wonderful!

The green-tinted oil gained favor only after the tree was brought to Bergamot, Italy, in the fifteenth century. There it was used to treat fevers, malaria, and intestinal worms. It now is also grown in the warm climates of California, Florida, and the Caribbean. According to legend, Christopher Columbus brought the tree to the Caribbean, where it was popularly used in voodoo practices to protect one from misfortune. Columbus may have had his own reasons for traveling with bergamot. Carrying the dried fruit in your pocket was thought to keep travelers safe on their journeys and soothe the stress of traveling.

Modern aromatherapists suggest placing a few drops of bergamot on a cloth and carrying it in your pocket or travel bag. Sniff the scented cloth while traveling to reduce stress, depression, anxiety, or insomnia.

PRINCIPAL CONSTITUENTS: Linalyl acetate, linalol, and up to 300 other components, including bergapten

SCENT: The fragrance is fresh, green, fruity, and cleanly refreshing, but slightly spicy and balsamic compared with other citruses. It mixes well with other scents, mellowing the overall fragrance while adding richness.

THERAPEUTIC PROPERTIES: Antiseptic, anti-inflammatory, antidepressant, antiviral, antibiotic

USED FOR: Bergamot fights several viruses, including those that cause flu, herpes, shingles, and chicken pox. Due to its versatile antibiotic properties, it also treats bacterial infections of the urinary system, mouth, and throat and a variety of skin conditions, including eczema. The best way to use it is diluted in a salve or massage oil that is applied externally over the afflicted area. As a natural deodorant, it not only provides a pleasant scent, but it kills bacteria that are responsible for odor. Add 30 drops to half a cup of cornstarch or arrowroot powder for body powder or ten drops per ounce to witch hazel solution from the drugstore for an instant deodorant. Bergamot is second only to lavender in its ability to relax brain waves when sniffed.

WARNINGS: Due to bergapten, bergamot can be photosensitizing, causing abnormal skin pigmentation when used externally by sensitive individuals who then go out in the sun. A bergapten-free essential oil is available; this should be noted on the bottle. While it may sound appealing to make your own Earl Grey tea, leave that up to the experts; they add only the tiniest amount of essential oil to the tea leaves in a quantity that is safe to ingest.

Birch

(Betula lenta)
Family: Betulaceae

The scent and flavor of birch has been a European and North American Indian favorite for centuries. Birch drinks were favored by those suffering from consumption because the natural aspirin, methyl salicylate, in the essential oil relieves pain and makes it easier to breathe. The essential oil was the closely guarded secret ingredient in the formula for the popular nineteenth-century men's fragrance "Russian Leather" — so named because the Russians used it to keep leather book bindings soft and free from insects and mold. European women scented their handkerchiefs in a perfume called Iceland Wintergreen that included birch and other essential oils. The North American birch was the actual source of the "wintergreen" essential oil. Although the two plants are not closely related botanically, they share similar chemistry, so they also have the same properties, fragrance, and the same familiar flavor found in gum, candies, beverages, and many medicines.

PRINCIPAL CONSTITUENTS: Methyl salicylate, creosol, guaiacol

SCENT: It has a clean, sweet, sharp, invigorating, and minty scent, like chewing gum.

THERAPEUTIC PROPERTIES: Astringent, antiseptic; promotes menstruation and alleviates joint pain

USED FOR: In a massage oil or liniment, birch can be rubbed over painful areas to ease muscular and arthritic pain and stiffness. Alternatively, a couple drops of birch essential oil, along with a drop or two of another oil such as lavender to soften birch's sharp scent, can be added to your bath for the same purpose. This type of aromatherapy bath is also useful to increase circulation and promote menstruation, especially when delayed by physical or emotional stress. A salve or lotion containing birch essential oil softens the roughness caused by psoriasis, eczema, and other skin problems. Add two drops per ounce to your hair conditioner to help prevent dandruff.

WARNINGS: Be sure not to overdo the suggested quantities of this potent essential oil, as it can be toxic in high doses. Since it smells like candy, store it safely away from children so they won't be tempted to taste it.

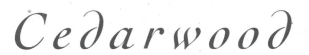

Cedarwood

(Cedrus deodora or C. atlantica)
Family: Cupressaceae

This majestic tree was used to build King
Solomon's temple because its fragrance was
thought to lead worshipers to prayer and
thus closer to God. The tree grows to 100
feet in height, lives more than 1,000 years,
and resists insect damage. The ancient Egyptians used cedar as a preservative and for
embalming, in cosmetics, and as incense.
More commonly, cedar is included in men's
colognes and aftershaves and is used to
make cigar boxes, cedar chests, and panel
closets. Cedar wood and its essential oil
make clothes smell great, and on a practical level, they repel wool moths. You won't
find true cedar of Lebanon oil because of
the shortage of trees, but Tibetan or Hi-
malayan cedarwood (*C. deodora*, meaning
"god tree"), and Atlas cedarwood (*C. atlantica*) have similar scents. The modern
source of most "cedarwood" oil is juniper
(*Juniperus virginiana*), known as "red cedar."
Don't confuse cedarwood with thuja or
cedar leaf (*Thuja occidentalis*).

PRINCIPAL CONSTITUENTS: Cedrene, cedrol, cedrenol, sometimes thujopsene, and others

SCENT: True cedar has a camphoraceous top note with a woodsy, balsamic undertone. Red cedar is sharper, like a freshly sharpened pencil.

THERAPEUTIC PROPERTIES: Antiseptic, astringent; brings on menstruation, clears mucus, sedates nerves, and stimulates circulation

USED FOR: Inhale the steam of cedarwood essential oil to treat respiratory infections and clear congestion. Add a few drops to a sitz bath to ease the pain and irritation of urinary infections and to cure the infection more quickly. Applied to oily skin, cedarwood essential oil is an astringent that dries and helps clear acne. Incorporate it into a facial wash, spritzer, or other cosmetic (10 drops of essential oil per ounce of preparation). Added to a salve (15 drops of essential oil per ounce of salve), it relieves dermatitis and, in some cases, eczema and psoriasis. For bites and itching, mix cedarwood and an equal part of alcohol or vegetable oil, and dab directly on the area. Add two drops of essential oil to every ounce of shampoo or hair conditioner to ease dandruff and possibly slow hair loss.

WARNINGS: Both cedar and juniper are best avoided during pregnancy. Tibetan cedar (*C. deodora*) is considered the safest.

Chamomile

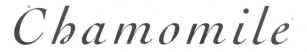

German (Matricaria recutita)
Family: Asteraceae (Compositae)

Chamomile's flowers resemble tiny daisies, but one sniff will have you thinking of apples instead. The herb has long been grown for its healing properties. Its smell was thought to relieve depression and to encourage relaxation. Medieval monks planted raised garden beds of chamomile, and those who were sad or depressed lay on them as therapy. Chamomile also was once a "strewing herb," spread on bare floors so that the scent was released when people walked on it. Drinking chamomile tea made from the flowers stimulates appetite before meals; after meals it settles the stomach. Roman chamomile *(Camaemelum nobile,* formerly *Anthemis nobilis)* yields a pale yellow essential oil that is an anti-inflammatory. When German chamomile is distilled, a chemical reaction produces the deep blue-green chamazulene that is even more potent an anti-inflammatory.

PRINCIPAL CONSTITUENTS: Esters of angelic and tiglic acids with pinene, farnesol, nerolidol, chamazulene, pinocarvone, and cineol

SCENT: The odor is sweet, applelike, and herbaceous.

THERAPEUTIC PROPERTIES: Anti-inflammatory, antiseptic; promotes digestion, relieves gas and nausea, encourages menstruation, soothes nervous tension, and promotes sleep

USED FOR: Inhaling chamomile tea's aroma relaxes both mind and body. Research studies show that chamomile relaxes emotions, muscles, and even brain waves. It eases the emotional ups and downs of PMS, menopause, and hyperactivity in children. It also helps control the pain of bruises, stiff joints, headaches, sore muscles, menstrual and digestive system cramping, as well as the pain and swelling of sprains and some allergic reactions. Chamomile is mild enough to ease a baby's colic and calm it for sleep. It is especially soothing in a massage oil, as a compress, or in a bath. Make a chamomile room spray by diluting 12 drops of the essential oil per ounce of distilled water. Chamomile is suitable for most complexion types or skin problems, from burns and eczema to varicose veins. It is especially useful for sensitive, puffy, or inflamed conditions. Add it to shampoos to lighten and brighten hair.

Cinnamon

(Cinnamomum zeylanicum)
Family: Lauraceae

The simple powder used in cooking starts off as the dry inner bark of a large 20-to-30-foot tree most likely growing in Sri Lanka (formerly Ceylon). The Arabs, who first brought cinnamon to the West, created a myth to frighten away rival traders, saying it could only be gathered in marshes from the nest of the great phoenix that was guarded by winged serpents and bats! The Portuguese finally seized Ceylon in 1505, but the plants were such coveted commodities that the Dutch later conquered the country, followed by the British in 1798. Then, as now, cinnamon flavored mouthwashes, foods, and drinks and was used as an aphrodisiac. Cinnamon's scent also stirs the appetite, invigorates and "warms" the senses, and may even produce a feeling of joy. There are several types of cinnamon oil to choose from: Oil can be distilled from the leaf or the much more potent bark, or you can obtain cassia oil, a less expensive relative of cinnamon that comes from China.

PRINCIPAL CONSTITUENTS: The more irritant bark is 40–50 percent cinnamaldehyde and 4–10 percent eugenol; the leaf is 3 percent cinnamaldehyde and 70–90 percent eugenol. Cinnamon also contains linalol, methylamine ketone, and others.

SCENT: It has a sweet, spicy-hot fragrance.

THERAPEUTIC PROPERTIES: Antiseptic, digestive, antiviral; relieves muscle spasms and rheumatic pain when used topically

USED FOR: In general, cinnamon is used as a physical and emotional stimulant. Researchers have found that it reduces drowsiness, irritability, and the pain and number of headaches. In one study, the aroma of cinnamon in the room helped participants to concentrate and perform better. The essential oil and its fragrance help relax tight muscles, ease painful joints, and relieve menstrual cramps. In addition, it increases circulation and sweating when used as a liniment. Use 2 to 4 drops per ounce of vegetable oil for a warming oil or 8 drops per ounce to make a hot liniment.

WARNINGS: Both bark and leaf oils can irritate mucous membranes, but the bark oil is especially hot. Use no more than one-half drop in the bath, and avoid its use in cosmetics since it can redden and even burn the skin.

Clary Sage

(Salvia sclarea)
Family: Lamiaceae

In ancient times, clary sage was praised as a panacea with the ability to render man immortal. Clary sage's name is derived from the Latin word *clarus*, meaning "clear." The tea was once thought not only to clear eyesight and the brain, but also to clarify one's intuition and allow one to see more clearly into the future. Simply sniffing the oil before going to bed can produce dramatic dreams and, when you awake, a euphoric state of mind. Clary was an important ingredient in one of the most popular European cordials. Along with elderflowers, it still flavors high quality Muscatel wine and Italian vermouth. Distilled from the flowering tops and leaves of a three-foot-tall perennial, clary sage now is produced mostly for flavoring a large variety of foods. In fact, the largest U.S. grower does not produce clary sage for aromatherapy purposes. It produces the herb for R. J. Reynolds, the tobacco company, which uses it to flavor cigarettes.

PRINCIPAL CONSTITUENTS: Linalyl acetate, linalol, pinene, myrcene, and phellandrene

SCENT: Similar to ambergris, it has a nutty, winelike character that is bittersweet, thick, and heady.

THERAPEUTIC PROPERTIES: Antidepressant, anti-inflammatory, astringent, sedative, deodorant; decreases gas and indigestion, brings on menstruation, relaxes muscles and nerves, and lowers blood pressure

USED FOR: Added to a massage oil or used in a compress, clary sage eases muscle and nervous tension and pain. Its relaxing action can reduce muscle spasms and asthma attacks and lower blood pressure. Especially good for female ailments, it helps one cope better with menstrual cramps or PMS and has established itself as a premier remedy for menopausal hot flashes. It may be a gentle hormonal stimulant. Improve your complexion by adding it to creams, especially if you have acne or thin, wrinkled, or inflamed skin. In Europe, a tea prepared from clary sage leaf soothes a sore throat.

WARNINGS: Large amounts can cause giddiness and headaches and raise blood pressure. Do not use with alcohol or if you are pregnant or suffer from breast cysts, uterine fibroids, or other estrogen-related disorders.

Clove

(Syzygium aromaticum)
Family: Myrtaceae

In ancient China, courtiers at the Han court held cloves in their mouths to freshen their breath before they had an audience with the emperor. Today, cloves are still used to sweeten breath. Modern dental preparations numb tooth and gum pain and quell infection with clove essential oil or its main constituent, eugenol. Simply inhaling the fragrance was once said to improve eyesight and fend off the plague. Clove's scent developed a reputation, now backed by science, for being stimulating. The fragrance was also believed to be an aphrodisiac. Cloves were so valuable that a Frenchman risked his life to steal a clove tree from the Dutch colonies in Indonesia and plant it in French ground. Once established, the slender evergreen trees bear buds for at least a century. The familiar clove buds used to poke hams and flavor mulled wine are picked while still unripe and dried before being shipped or distilled into essential oil.

PRINCIPAL CONSTITUENTS: Eugenol, eugenyl acetate, caryophyllene

SCENT: The fragrance is powerful, sweet-spicy, and hot, with fruity top notes.

THERAPEUTIC PROPERTIES: Antibacterial, antifungal, antihistamine; decreases gas and indigestion, clears mucous from the lungs, expels intestinal worms

USED FOR: As an antiseptic and pain-reliever, clove essential oil relieves toothaches, flu, colds, and bronchial congestion. But don't try to use it straight on a baby's gums for teething as is often suggested, or you may end up with a screaming baby because it tastes so strong and hot. Instead mix only two drops of clove bark oil in at least a teaspoon of vegetable oil. It can still be hot, however, so try it in your own mouth first. Then apply it directly to the baby's gums. In a heating liniment, clove essential oil helps sore muscles and arthritis. Mix 30 drops of clove essential oil in one ounce of apple cider vinegar, shake well, and dab on athlete's foot. Researchers have found that the spicy aroma of clove reduces drowsiness, irritability, and headaches.

WARNINGS: The essential oil irritates skin and mucous membranes, so be sure to dilute it before use. Clove leaf is almost pure eugenol; do not use it in aromatherapy preparations.

Cypress

(Cupressus sempervirens)

Family: Cupressaceae

The landscapes of southern France and Greece are graced with this statuesque evergreen, which first came from the island of Cyprus where it was worshiped as a representation of the goddess Beruth. The tree appears in art and literature as an emblem of generation, death, the immortal soul, and woe. This long association with mortality continues today, for modern Egyptians use cypress wood for coffins, while the French and Americans plant it in graveyards. Greeks say that cypress clears the mind during stressful times and comforts mourners. Cypress stanches bleeding (Hippocrates recommended it for hemorrhoids) and the Chinese chewed its small cones, rich in essential oils and astringents, to heal bleeding gums. The Chinese also revered cypress, but associated it with contemplation because its roots grow in the form of a seated man. The greenish essential oil is distilled from the tree's needles or twigs and sometimes from its cones.

PRINCIPAL CONSTITUENTS: Pinene, camphene, sylvestrene, cymene, sabinol

SCENT: It has a smoky, pungent, pinelike, and spicy scent.

THERAPEUTIC PROPERTIES: Antiseptic, astringent, deodorant; relieves rheumatic pain, relaxes muscle spasms and cramping, stops bleeding, and constricts blood vessels.

USED FOR: Cypress's specialty is treating circulation problems, such as low blood pressure, poor circulation, varicose veins, and hemorrhoids. Because it helps heal broken capillaries and also discourages fluid retention, it is a favored essential oil at menopause. For these uses, add 8 drops to every ounce of cream or lotion and apply gently to the afflicted region a couple of times a day. You can also alleviate laryngitis, spasmodic coughing, and lung congestion just by putting a drop on your pillow. A European folk remedy is to inhale smoke from the burning gum resin to relieve sinus congestion, although inhaling a few drops of the essential oil in steam is a healthier approach. Place a cypress compress over the abdomen to quell excessive menstruation, urinary infection, or inflammation. Because of its astringent, antiseptic, and deodorant properties, dilute about 6 drops of cypress essential oil in vinegar or aloe vera for an oily complexion or to reduce excessive sweating.

Eucalyptus

(Eucalyptus globulus)

Family: Myrtaceae

Australia's "blue forests" are named for the haze produced by the tree's essential oil. When you walk through the groves, the blue mist that mutes the surrounding scenery can be almost intoxicating. One can't help but take deep breaths of its refreshing scent — which is perhaps why aromatherapists use it to "clear the air," helping to resolve disagreements in interpersonal conflicts.

Eucalyptus or "gum" trees originated in Australia and Tasmania, but they are now found in subtropical regions all over the globe. They are one of the tallest and fastest growing trees. The eucalyptus tree was introduced at the Paris Exposition in 1867 after the director of the botanical gardens in Melbourne, Australia, suggested that the essential oil might be an antiseptic replacement for cajeput oil. He was right. The French government then planted the fast-growing trees in Algeria to ward off the "noxious gases" thought to be responsible for malaria. It worked, but ironically this was not due to the essential oil, but because the water-hungry trees transformed the marsh into dry land, eliminating the mosquitos' habitat.

Eucalyptus' thick, long, bluish-green leaves are distilled to provide essential oil. Blue gum eucalyptus, the most widely cultivated variety, provides most of the commercially available oil, although with more than 600 species, there are a variety of scents. Aromatherapists sometimes favor the more relaxing qualities and pleasant scent of the lemony *E. citriodora.*

A very inexpensive oil, eucalyptus is used liberally to scent aftershaves and colognes and as an antiseptic in mouthwashes and household cleansers.

PRINCIPAL CONSTITUENTS: Cineol or eucalyptol, pinene, limonene, and at least 250 other compounds. Varieties can include citronellal, cineole, cryptone, piperitone.

SCENT: The odor is pungent, sharp, and somewhat camphoraceous.

THERAPEUTIC PROPERTIES: Antibacterial, antiviral, deodorant; clears mucous from the lungs; as a liniment, relieves rheumatic, arthritic, and other types of pain

USED FOR: Highly antiseptic, eucalyptus has long been a household remedy in Australia for treating everything from flu, fever, and sore throat to skin and muscle pain. Most liniments and vapor rubs contain it or eucalyptol, one of its principal constituents. It is the most popular essential oil steam for relieving sinus and lung congestion such as asthma. Inhale the steam as described on page 73, add one or two drops of oil to a compress, or put three or four drops in your bath. Especially appropriate for skin eruptions and oily complexions, it is also used for acne, herpes, and chicken pox. For a homemade preparation, mix eucalyptus essential oil with an equal amount of apple cider vinegar and dab on problem areas. This mix can also be used as an antiseptic on wounds, boils, and insect bites. The scent increases brain wave activity and counters physical and mental fatigue. Carry eucalyptus with you on long car trips, or smell it to help you study. International Flavors and Fragrances, Inc., a research and development corporation in New Jersey, found that sniffing eucalyptus increases your energy.

WARNINGS: Do not use during an asthma attack.

F i r

(Abies alba; species such as Pinus and Picea)
Family: Pinaceae

The balsam fir, a native of northern Europe, is our well-known Christmas tree. To the Irish Celts it was a tree of birth and thus it signified the birth of the new year, and so the original "Yule logs" were probably fir. For centuries, boughs were scattered over floors of churches and houses during winter, providing a clean, scented covering. Perhaps long ago, people realized that the uplifting fragrance helped overcome winter blues and encouraged feelings of contentment and joy. This use of fir is reflected in Greek myth. When the god Attis was about to die from a wound, Cybele turned him into a fir so that he would remain "evergreen." Fir essential oil is distilled from the twigs or needles of many different conifers, including spruces and pines, yielding a rich variety of fragrances. The Canadian Balsam (*A. balsamea*) and Siberian Fir (*A. siberica*) have an especially pleasant, forestlike scent. In comparison, the scent of pine essential oil is sharper. The harsher turpentine oil also comes from members of the pine family and is used in varnishes and paints, preservatives, and lamp oil. For general purposes, all of these essential oils have highly antiseptic properties.

PRINCIPAL CONSTITUENTS: Santene, pinene, limonehe, bornyl acetate, lauraldehyde

SCENT: Similar to that of Christmas trees, it is fresh, softly balsamic, invigorating, and forestlike.

THERAPEUTIC PROPERTIES: Antibacterial, deodorant; relieves pain and coughing, clears mucous from the lungs, kills mold

USED FOR: Fir and pine essential oils soothe muscle and rheumatism pain and increase poor circulation when used in a massage oil or when added to a liniment or bath. They also help prevent bronchial and urinary infections and reduce coughing, including that caused by bronchitis and asthma. The best ways to utilize the essential oil are either through inhalation or via a chest rub. It is occasionally added to a salve or other skin preparation as an antiseptic for skin infections. Pine and fir stimulate energy, according to research from International Flavors and Fragrances, Inc., in New Jersey. An aromatherapy alarm clock from Japan uses the forest scent of pine or fir along with eucalyptus for its wake-up call.

Frankincense

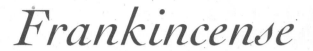

(Boswellia carteri)
Family: *Berseraceae*

The frankincense burned as church incense today is the same as that used by ancient peoples who inhabited the Middle East and North Africa. Eventually the use of frankincense spread throughout Europe and eastward into India, and it was burned as an offering to the gods of many cultures. It was one of the four "sweet scents" used by Jews in their ceremonial incense, and it was presented each Sabbath day with the shewbread. For Christians it was one of the three precious gifts brought by the Magi to the infant Jesus.

Exceeding the value of precious metals and gems, frankincense was only produced by 3,000 families called *Sabians* from the land of Punt. The men chosen to prune and gather frankincense gum had to undergo ritual purification. Frankincense was so greatly valued because its fragrance was believed to heighten spirituality, sending one into a deep, meditative relaxation that enhanced worship. Aromatherapists and massage practitioners have observed that frank-incense's fragrance does deepen breathing, aid relaxation, and cause the lungs to expand. Modern science backs up these observations by showing that, when burned, frankincense releases molecules of trahydrocannabinole, a psychoactive compound that may be responsible for uplifting the spirit.

Charred and powdered, frankincense was the major ingredient in the traditional black kohl that Egyptian women still wear as eyeliner. It was believed to help women see a more spiritual aspect of the world, to avoid ill-fate, and to prevent eye infection. Of course, it has been, and still is, used in expensive perfume.

This small tree has been planted on rocky hill-sides in Yemen and Oman, but the highest quality frankincense still comes from North Africa, with some produced in Somalia, China, and India. The clear to pale yellow oil is steam distilled from hard "tears" of oleo gum resin.

PRINCIPAL CONSTITUENTS: Olibanol, resinous matter, and terpenes

SCENT: The fragrance is soft, balsamic, and sometimes lemony or camphorous.

THERAPEUTIC PROPERTIES: Antiseptic, anti-inflammatory, antifungal, astringent, seda-tive; clears lung congestion, decreases gas and indigestion, brings on menstruation

USED FOR: Historically, it has been utilized for treating syphilis, infections, and all kinds of skin disorders. Ayurvedic medicine from India has long suggested its use on inflamed skin conditions. Its antiseptic and skin-healing properties fight bacterial and fungal skin infections and boils. Since it's quite expensive, however, it is usually reserved for the most difficult cases, such as unsightly scars that remain after an infection has healed, and hard-to-heal wounds. For problem skin areas, use a couple drops of frankincense in an equal amount of vegetable oil. Frankincense is excellent on mature skin and acne. It is especially good when middle-aged women experience those conditions and also want to prevent wrinkles. Make a compress or massage oil with frankincense for breast cysts or for infection of the lungs, reproductive organs, or urinary tract. It also increases menstrual flow.

Geranium

(Pelargonium graveoloens)
Family: Geraniaceae

In experimental outpatient clinics in Azerbaijan, patients sit comfortably in an aromatherapy room sniffing fragrant plants such as rose geranium. They inhale the aromas according to a prescription, which specifies how many times a week and for how many minutes the fragrance should be inhaled. According to the clinic, inhaling geranium actually lowers or raises blood pressure a few points, depending upon what the person's body requires. They also report success in using geranium to control depression and mental disturbances.

A relative newcomer to the fragrance trade, geranium is a small, tender, South African perennial whose essential oil was not distilled until the nineteenth century. Since it is a veritable medicine cabinet with a lovely scent, it became an instant hit. It is also an insect repellent, and one that is certainly more aromatically pleasing than the commonly used citronella. The scent of geranium mixes well with almost any other essential oil. There are more than 600 varieties, including several with a roselike fragrance. The pharmaceutical industry uses its main component, geraniol, to stretch true rose oil or, with other components, to make a synthetic rose.

PRINCIPAL CONSTITUENTS: Geraniol, citronellol, linalol, borneol, terpineol, and many others

SCENT: The scent is bright, with a herbaceous-rose-citrus combination.

THERAPEUTIC PROPERTIES: Antidepressant, antiseptic, astringent; stops bleeding, possibly gently stimulates the adrenals and normalizes hormones

USED FOR: In its native Africa, geranium was used as an herb tea to stop diarrhea and internal bleeding. A popular skin therapy, the essential oil treats a host of problems including inflammation, eczema, acne, burns, infected wounds, fungus (like ringworm), lice, shingles, and herpes. It also decreases scarring and stretch marks. Use it in the form of a salve, cream, lotion, or massage/body oil, whichever is most appropriate. It balances all complexion types and is said to delay wrinkling. Inhale this pleasant scent to treat PMS, menopause, fluid retention, and other hormone-related problems, or include it in body rubs and baths.

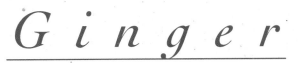

Ginger

(Zingiber officinale)
Family: Zingiberaceae

You have certainly encountered ginger's succulent, spicy rhizome in the grocery store. Used fresh, or dried and powdered for a culinary spice, it flavors ginger ale, cakes, and cookies and is a major ingredient in curries and other Eastern cuisines. The Chinese scholar Confucius ate fresh ginger with every meal. Since it was one of the earliest herbs transported in the spice trade, it is now difficult to determine if ginger originated in India or China. One ancient Indian trading city was named *Shunthi*, the Sanskrit name for ginger.

From 200 B.C.E. and continuing for a thousand years, Arab traders monopolized the ginger trade, carrying the root in sealed earthenware jars on camel caravans through Asia Minor or on boats sailing through the Arabian Sea to Egypt. Ginger was also used in ancient Greece, Rome, and even Britain before the Norman conquest. Spanish conquistadors introduced ginger to the West Indies. In the Philippines, ginger is used to fish with as it is believed to attract fish. It is also thought to drive out the evil spirits that cause disease. In Melanesia, men used it to win the affection of women; Arabs consider it an aphrodisiac that greatly increases energy. Could St. Hildegarde of Bingen have known this in the twelfth century when she recommended its use for stimulating the vigor of older men married to young women? Or perhaps she was aware that its name comes from the same root as "generate" and "beget," meaning to procreate? Because of such qualities, the word "ginger" has developed an informal meaning of liveliness and vigor.

PRINCIPAL CONSTITUENTS: Gingerin, gingenol, gingerone, zingiberene, linalol, camphene, other alcohols and terpenes, with citral and resins

SCENT: It smells peppery sharp, pungent, aromatic, and warm, sometimes with a camphoraceous or lemon note.

THERAPEUTIC PROPERTIES: Stimulates circulation, increases perspiration, relieves gas and pain, aids digestion

USED FOR: Ginger stimulates the appetite and relieves inflammation throughout the body. An ancient Ayurvedic remedy from India advises placing crushed ginger rhizome on the forehead for a headache. You can use this ancient headache treatment or a more simple modern version by adding a few drops of ginger essential oil to water, soaking a cloth in it, and using it as a compress. Also use a ginger compress wrapped around the neck or placed on the chest to ease sore throat or lung congestion. The smell of it alone will often open congested sinuses. If you experience nausea or motion sickness, inhale a drop placed on a hankie, eat a little candied ginger, or sip ginger ale, which contains a small amount of the essential oil. To relieve indigestion or menstrual cramps, rub a massage oil containing ginger into the skin on your abdomen or place a poultice made from the grated root on it. In a warming liniment, ginger essential oil treats poor circulation and sore or cramped muscles, since it decreases the substances in the body that make muscles cramp. Drinking ginger tea made by boiling the fresh rhizome for about twenty minutes is a classic cold, cough, and fever treatment (try adding a little lemon juice, chopped garlic, maple syrup, and cayenne). Ginger tea can also be an energizing substitute for coffee in the mornings.

Jasmine

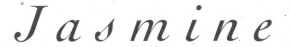

(Jasminum officinalis and J. grandiflorum)
Family: Oleaceae

Probably an Iranian native, jasmine, whose name means "heavenly felicity," has captured the imagination of poets and perfumers for thousands of years. In China it was used to scent and flavor jasmine tea.

The small white flowers of this vinelike evergreen shrub, with their intriguing, complex scent, are intensely fragrant and found in most great perfumes. Jasmine is also known as "mistress of the night" and "moonlight of the grove" because its seductive scent reaches its peak late at night. Even the production of the essential oil is exotic. The flowers are gathered at night, when they produce the most oil, and laid on a layer of fat for the method of extraction called enfleurage. It is first made into a concrete, which is solid, then the fat is separated to leave an absolute. Try as chemists might to make it, the scent cannot be duplicated. Synthetic jasmine is so harsh, it demands a touch of the true essential oil to soften it.

PRINCIPAL CONSTITUENTS: Ketone jasmone, alpha terpineol, benzyl acetate, benzyl alcohol, indol, linalol, linalyl acetate, phenylacetic acid, farnesol, and many more

SCENT: It has a distinctively rich, warm floral fragrance that is sweetly exotic, with a fruity-tea undertone.

THERAPEUTIC PROPERTIES: Antidepressant; relaxes nerves, relieves muscle spasms and cramping

USED FOR: Jasmine sedates the nervous system, so it is good for jangled nerves, headaches, insomnia, and depression and for taking the emotional edge off PMS and menopause, although keep in mind its age-old reputation as an aphrodisiac! Studies at Toho University School of Medicine in Tokyo show that jasmine also enhances mental alertness and stimulates brain waves. In another study, it was able to help computer operators reduce by one-third the number of mistakes they made. It also eases muscle cramping, such as menstrual cramps. Cosmetically, the oil is wonderful for sensitive or mature skin. In its native India, jasmine flowers infused into sesame oil are applied to abscesses and sores that are difficult to heal. A similar preparation can be made by adding 2 drops of jasmine essential oil to 1 ounce vegetable oil.

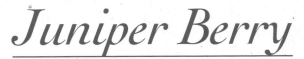

Juniper Berry

(Juniperus communis)
Family: *Cupressaceae*

Gin was named after *genièvre*, the French word for juniper berry, which gives gin its characteristic flavor. The British said that an infusion of berries could restore lost youth; however, juniper's more important role was for protection. It traditionally was planted at the entrance of homes to guard against evil and ghosts. Burning the branches was found to ward off contagious diseases, so medieval physicians chewed the berries while on duty and burned the branches in hospitals. In World War II, the French returned to burning juniper in hospitals as an antiseptic when their supply of drugs ran low. Fresh berries offer the highest quality oil, but needles, branches, and berries that have already been distilled to flavor gin are sometimes used. Everyone is familiar with the lively scent of juniper wood because it is used for making pencils (see Cedar). With many of the same properties as cedarwood, it also acts as a wool moth repellent.

PRINCIPAL CONSTITUENTS: Pinene, myrcene, sabinene, limonene, cymene, borneol, camphene, juniperine, terpenic alcohol, and terpineol

SCENT: The fragrance is pungent, herbaceous, peppery, pinelike, and camphorous. The needles produce a turpentinelike scent called juniper tar.

THERAPEUTIC PROPERTIES: Antiseptic, astringent; relieves the aches of rheumatism, arthritis, and sore muscles; increases urination and circulation; encourages menstruation; aids digestion

USED FOR: Juniper berry essential oil is used in massage oils, liniments, and baths to treat arthritic and rheumatic pain, varicose veins, hemorrhoids, fluid retention (especially before menstruation), and bladder infection. Inhale it in a steam to relieve bronchial congestion, infection, and bronchial spasms. Inhalation may also lift your spirits, as sniffing the oil seems to work as a pick-me-up and to counter general debility. Cosmetically it is suitable for acne complexions and eczema. Add approximately 6 drops per ounce to shampoos for greasy hair or dandruff.

WARNINGS: Juniper can overstimulate the kidneys, so do not use it when they are inflamed or infected. Inflamed or infected kidneys can be very serious, so be sure to seek a doctor's advice.

Lavender

(Lavandula angustifolia)
Family: Lamiaceae (Labiatae)

A well-loved Mediterranean herb, lavender has been associated with cleanliness since Romans first added it to their bathwater. In fact, the name comes from the Latin *lavandus*, meaning to wash. A Christian legend says that lavender originally had no odor, but since the Virgin Mary dried Jesus' swaddling clothes on it, it has had a heavenly perfume. Today lavender remains a favorite for scenting clothing and closets, soaps, and even furniture polish. Lavender was traditionally inhaled to ease exhaustion, insomnia, irritability, and depression. In the Victorian era, women revived themselves from faints caused by tight corsets with lavender-filled swooning pillows. Two related plants called spike (*L. latifolia*) and lavandin (*L. intermedia*) are produced in greater quantities; but they are more camphorous and harsher in scent, with inferior healing properties, although they are useful for disinfecting. Less expensive to produce, they are commonly sold as lavender.

PRINCIPAL CONSTITUENTS: Linalol, linalyl acetate, geranyle, eucalyptol, pinene, limonene, cineole, phenol, coumarins, flavonoids

SCENT: The aroma is sweet, floral, and herbal with balsamic undertones.

THERAPEUTIC PROPERTIES: Antiseptic, circulatory stimulant; relieves muscle spasms and cramping

USED FOR: Lavender is among the safest and most widely used of all aromatherapy oils. It relieves muscle pain, migraines and other headaches, and inflammation. It is also one of the most antiseptic essential oils, treating many types of infection, including lung, sinus, vaginal, and especially candida infections. Lavender is suitable for all skin types. Cosmetically, it appears to be a cell regenerator. It prevents scarring and stretch marks and reputedly slows the development of wrinkles. It is used on burns, sun-damaged skin, wounds, rashes, and, of course, skin infections. Lavender also treats indigestion, including colic, and boosts immunity. Of several fragrances tested by aromatherapy researchers, lavender was most effective at relaxing brain waves and reducing stress. It also reduced computer errors by almost one-fourth when used to scent the office.

L e m o n

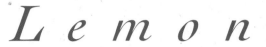

(Citrus limonum)
Family: Rutaceae

The lemon tree hails from Asia, but has been cultivated in Italy since at least the fourth century. It is now grown throughout the Mediterranean, Australia, Central and South America, California, and Florida.

Most people would immediately describe lemon as having a "clean" smelling fragrance. As a result, it is used in a vast number of household cleaning products that are advertised as "lemon-fresh" and "sparkling." Aromatherapists use the tie-in with cleanliness to help people purge feelings of imperfection and impurity and to build up their confidence. Lemon essential oil is a major ingredient in commercial beverages, foods, and pharmaceuticals, although the cheaper lemongrass or even synthetic citral is often added to stretch it. It also is popular for its fresh aroma in cologne and many cosmetics, especially cleansing creams and lotions.

The flowers are occasionally distilled for their pleasant aroma, but cold pressing the peel produces the essential oil that you are most likely to find. Like other citruses, the oil keeps well for only about a year; so you can prolong its life by storing it in a cool place or even in the refrigerator.

PRINCIPAL CONSTITUENTS: Limonene (up to 90 percent), terpinene, pinenes, sabinene, myrcene, citral, linalol, geraniol, citronellal, bergamotene, and others

SCENT: Distinctively clean, sharp, and citrus, the fragrance has a smoother, creamier aroma in the higher qualities.

THERAPEUTIC PROPERTIES: Antiseptic, antidepressant, antiviral; decreases indigestion, stops bleeding

USED FOR: Made into a hot drink with maple sugar or honey, the lemon fruit and peel have soothed colds, fevers, sore throat, and coughs throughout the world for centuries. Studies show that the oil increases the activity of the immune system by stimulating the production of the white corpuscles that fight infection. Additionally, lemon essential oil counters a wide range of viral and bacterial infections. Massage it on the skin in a vegetable oil base to relieve congested lymph glands. Inhaled it has been shown to reduce blood pressure. Since it also reduces water retention and increases mineral absorption, it can be helpful in achieving weight loss. Incorporated into cosmetics, lemon is best used on oily complexions and to clean acne, blackheads, and other skin impurities. In Japan the essential oil is diffused through the air systems of offices and factories because it increases concentration and the ability to memorize and noticeably reduces mistakes. Research confirms that the aroma of lemon is relaxing to brain waves, which improves concentration. It was the most effective essential oil tested in reducing computer errors; those working in a lemon-scented room made less than half the mistakes of those working in unscented rooms. Because it seems to stimulate the mind while calming emotions, sniffing lemon can be helpful when making decisions.

WARNINGS: The essential oil of lemon is occasionally photosensitizing for very sensitive people; that is, wearing a skin product containing it during exposure to the sun could cause a skin reaction. However, this reaction is very uncommon.

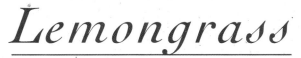

Lemongrass

(Cymbopogon citratus)
Family: Poaceae (Gramineae)

What gives Ivory Soap its familiar scent? The not-so-familiar lemongrass. A fast-growing, tall perennial grass originally from India and Sri Lanka, lemongrass found its way into traditional cuisines throughout Southeast Asia. It is used extensively in Thai fish soups and curries and is seen more and more frequently in supermarkets in North America.

An important medicinal and culinary herb in South and Central America, South East Asia, and the Caribbean, it is widely known as "fever grass." India's Ayurvedic medical tradition, for instance, has long used it to treat cholera and fevers. A relatively inexpensive essential oil, it's often the source of the lemon scent found in cosmetics and hair preparations. Its pleasant, clean fragrance is also incorporated into soaps, perfumes, and deodorants, and it flavors many canned and frozen foods. No wonder it is one of the ten best-selling essential oils in the world.

Along with related oils such as the lemon-rose scented palmarosa (*C. martini*) and citronella (*C. nardus*), it often adulterates more costly essential oils like melissa and lemon verbena to stretch them. Palmarosa is frequently used in skin preparations, while citronella is well known as an insect repellent and cleanser. The yellow to amber oil of these grasses is distilled from their partially dried leaves.

PRINCIPAL CONSTITUENTS: Citral (up to 85 percent), myrcene, citronellol, dipentene, farnesol, furfurol, geraniol, and many more

SCENT: The scent is lemon/herbal, grassy, and slightly bitter. Palmarosa has a pleasant rose scent. Citronella is very lemony.

THERAPEUTIC PROPERTIES: Antiseptic, deodorant, astringent; relieves rheumatic and other pain, relaxes nerves

USED FOR: In traditional medicine, lemongrass is usually given in the form of a tea or foot bath made from the fresh herb, from which the patient additionally benefits by inhaling the scent. Lemongrass also treats pain arising from indigestion, rheumatism, and nerve conditions. Researchers also found this refreshing fragrance to reduce headaches and irritability and to prevent drowsiness. To make a foot bath, add about 3 drops of lemongrass oil to 2 or 3 quarts of warm water in a small tub. Stir well and keep your feet in the water for at least 20 minutes. You can also add a few drops to your bath. Lemongrass is an antiseptic suitable for use on various types of skin infections, usually as a wash or compress, and is especially effective on ringworm and infected sores. In fact, studies found that it is more effective against staph infection than either penicillin or streptomycin. When added to a hair conditioner, facial water, or vinegar, it counters oily hair and acne by decreasing oil production. Add 12 drops of the essential oil per ounce of apple cider vinegar and dab or spray on the afflicted area. You can spray this same solution in the air, on a counter top, or along walls and floors to discourage insect invasions and mold. Add it to pet shampoos as a bug repellent.

WARNINGS: It is nontoxic, but causes skin sensitivity in some people.

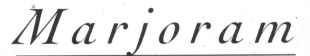

Marjoram

(Origanum marjorana)
Family: Lamiaceae (Labiatae)

"Sweet marjoram" is a low, bushy perennial native to Asia but naturalized in Europe, where singers learned to preserve and strengthen their voices with the honeyed tea. Traditionally it was given to those who felt unstable, physically debilitated, or irritable. Ancient Greeks planted the herb on their ancestors' graves to ensure them a peaceful sleep. The Romans said that the goddess Venus used marjoram to cure her son Eros' wounds and that it was scentless until she touched it. Marjoram is probably what is called "hyssop" in the Bible, where it is noted for personal cleansing and purification of the temples. Marjoram had a reputation for endowing longevity and was an antidote to serpent poison. The greenish-yellow oil is distilled from the plant's flowering tops. Its taste and properties are milder than the closely related oregano, which is so strong and potentially toxic that it is seldom used in aromatherapy.

PRINCIPAL CONSTITUENTS: Carvacrol, thymol, borneol, camphor, linalol, linalyl acetate, cineol, cymeme, sabinene, and terpineol

SCENT: The odor is sweet, herby, and pungent in concentration. When diluted, it mellows to an almost warm, spicy floral with a hint of camphor.

THERAPEUTIC PROPERTIES: Antioxidant; calms nerves, clears mucous from the lungs, relieves pain, improves digestion, brings on menstruation, lowers high blood pressure, stops bleeding

USED FOR: A good sedative, marjoram eases stiff joints and muscle spasms, including tics, excessive coughing, menstrual cramps, and headaches (especially migraines). It also slightly lowers high blood pressure. Testing has shown it to be one of the most effective fragrances in relaxing brain waves. As a result, it makes an excellent calming massage oil, delightful when combined with the softer lavender. Add a few drops to your bath to counter stress or insomnia. Since it has specific properties that fight the viruses and bacteria responsible for colds, flu, or laryngitis, add a few drops of essential oil to either a chest balm or bath, or put 2 or 3 drops in a bowl of hot water and inhale the steam. In healing salves and creams, it also soothes burns, bruises, and inflammation. Marjoram is also an antioxidant that naturally preserves food.

Myrrh

(Commiphora myrrha)

Family: Burseraceae

Myrrh has been used since antiquity as an incense to inspire prayer and meditation and to fortify the spirit. This small, scrubby, spiny tree from the semidesert regions of the Middle East and North East Africa is not very handsome, but it makes up for its looks with the precious gum it exudes. An important trade item for several thousand years, myrrh was a primary ingredient in ancient cosmetics and incenses. The Egyptians mummified their dead with it, while other cultures burned it in cremations. Believed to comfort sorrow, its name means "bitter tears." This may also refer to the bitter-tasting myrrh sap, which oozes in tear-like drops when the tree's bark is cut. Myrrh was added to wine by both the Greeks and Hebrews to heighten their sensual awareness. The yellow to amber-colored oil is distilled from the gum and frequently added to toothpastes and gum preparations to help alleviate mouth ulcers, gum inflammation, and infection.

PRINCIPAL CONSTITUENTS: Pinene, dipentene, heerabolene, limonene, cadinene, formic acid, acetic acid, myrrholic acid, eugenol, cinnamaldehyde, cuminaldehyde, plus resins

SCENT: It has a warm, spicy, bitter odor, with smoky and musky undertones.

THERAPEUTIC PROPERTIES: Antiseptic, anti-inflammatory, antibacterial and antifungal, decongestant, astringent; heals wounds, brings on menstruation

USED FOR: Myrrh is an expensive but effective treatment for chapped, cracked, or aged skin, eczema, bruises, infection, varicose veins, ringworm, and athlete's foot. Included in many ointments, it dries weepy wounds. It is a specific remedy for mouth and gum disease and is found in many oral preparations, as it fights candida infections such as thrush. It is very helpful applied on herpes sores and blisters: Add it to a lip balm, using about 25 drops per ounce. Lozenges or syrup containing myrrh treat coughs. As an additional bonus, it increases the activity of the immune system. Herbalists and aromatherapists use myrrh to gradually regulate an overactive thyroid. It can also increase menstrual flow.

WARNINGS: Due to a possible increase of thyroid activity, do not use myrrh if you have an overactive thyroid.

Neroli

(Citrus aurantium)
Family: Rutaceae

An Indochina native, the bitter orange produces the blossoms used for an oil known to aromatherapists and perfumers as neroli. The trees are grown commercially in France, Morocco, Tunisia, and Egypt and are quite different from the sweet orange that produces orange oil. One story is that neroli was named after a sixteenth century princess from Nerola, Italy, who loved the orange blossom scent. This scent, which is considered intensely female, became a symbol of purity, chastity, and eternal love. Neroli was thought to influence creativity in other ways, especially in music and writing. Modern aromatherapists regard neroli more as a treatment for depression. The blossoms may be distilled, made into a concrete by enfleurage, or extracted with solvents to create an absolute. A by-product of distillation, "orange flower water," is used in cooking and as a skin toner. Neroli is the main ingredient of the original *eau de cologne*, which was used both as a body fragrance and as a skin toner. Neroli was also a favorite of Marie Antoinette as well as Napoleon, who was said to go through several bottles a day as an aftershave. Distilling the leaves and stems of the bitter orange produces an essential oil called petitgrain that is frequently used in men's cologne today and often adulterates the far more expensive neroli.

PRINCIPAL CONSTITUENTS: Nerol, nerolidol, geraniol, jasmone, dipentene, terpineol, farnesol, indol, l-camphene, pinene, acetic esters, and more

SCENT: The scent is bittersweet, floral, spicy, distinctive, and often unpleasantly strong until diluted.

THERAPEUTIC PROPERTIES: Sedative; relieves muscle spasms and cramping, stimulates circulation

USED FOR: Neroli's favored use is for circulation problems, especially hemorrhoids and high blood pressure. It makes a wonderfully fragrant and effective cosmetic for mature, dry, and sensitive skin and is also one of the best essential oils to add to a vaginal cream during menopause. It reputedly regenerates skin cells and has anti-aging properties. For the ultimate luxury, add it to your bath to ease tension from PMS, menopause, or life in general.

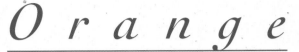

Orange

(Citrus sinensis)

Family: Rutaceae

Brought to the Mediterranean from Asia by the Saracens during the time of the crusades, the familiar sweet orange now comes from Sicily, Israel, Spain, and the U.S., each country's essential oil offering slightly different characteristics. They are rich in vitamins A, B, and C, flavonoids, and minerals. The Chinese, however, correctly warned in the *Chu-lu*—the first monograph describing the various citruses that was written in 1178—that they can increase lung congestion.

Oranges were considered symbols of fruitfulness, and the Greeks called them the "golden apple of the Hesperides." The god Zeus is said to have given an orange to his bride Hera at their wedding.

In 1290, Eleanor of Castile brought oranges to England, where they were grown as luxuries in greenhouses or "orangeries." In northern climates, only the very wealthy could afford oranges, and they were often given as extravagant gifts at Christmastime. In European courts they were stuck with cloves and carried as a pomander to dispel disagreeable odors and emotions such as depression and nervousness, as well as to bring more cheer into dreary winter days. The essential oil is cold pressed from the peel and lasts only about a year, so keep it cool and away from direct sunlight.

PRINCIPAL CONSTITUENTS: Limonene (up to 90 percent), with aldehydes, citral, citronellol, geraniol, linalol, methyl anthranilate, and terpineol

SCENT: It has a perky, lively, and distinctively orange scent. The related tangerine is brighter and sweeter, while petitgrain is harsher, sharper, and considerably more herby or "green."

THERAPEUTIC PROPERTIES: Sedative; relieves muscle spasms, cramping, and indigestion

USED FOR: Orange's greatest claim to aromatherapy fame is its ability to affect moods and to lower high blood pressure. In fact, just sniffing it lowers blood pressure a couple points. It is also a good adjunct treatment for irregular heartbeat. Research at International Flavors and Fragrances, Inc., in New Jersey found that orange also reduces anxiety. You don't even need to buy the essential oil; simply peel an orange and inhale its aroma. Although not as antibiotic as lemon, it still has some value in fighting flu, colds, and breaking up congested lymph, especially when added to massage oil. The aroma of oranges is a favorite of children, and they will usually be more enthusiastic about an aromatherapy treatment when it is included. Also use the massage oil to ease a bout of indigestion or overcome a light case of insomnia or depression. Cosmetically it is good for oily complexions, although essential oils with more sophisticated fragrances are preferred.

WARNINGS: The oil is only slightly photosensitizing, but still go easy in baths or any skin preparations since it can burn the skin — just 4 drops in a bathtub can be enough to irritate and redden sensitive skin. Related oils such as that of tangerine or mandarin (*C. reticulata*) are milder and safer choices for pregnant women and very young children.

Patchouli

(Pogostemon cablin)
Family: Lamiaceae

In India this essential oil with the lyrical name of *patcha pat* has long been used to keep moths and other insects out of linens and woolen shawls and rugs. It is the characteristic scent found in Indian bedspreads and cottons. Hand-woven silk and wool rugs from Persia, India, and Turkey had dried patchouli leaves laid on them before they were rolled for shipping. Europeans actually refused to buy cheaper local imitation Oriental rugs because they didn't smell authentic. To some people the scent of patchouli is exotic, sensual, and luxurious, but to others it's too forceful and repellent. It is so overpowering that most cosmetics forgo its virtues in favor of other essential oils that are more universally appealing. The leaves of this pretty Malaysian bush carry little indication of their potential, since the scent is only developed through oxidation. The leaves must be fermented and aged before being distilled, which can take as long as 24 hours. Even then, the translucent yellow oil smells harsh. As it ages, it develops patchouli's distinctive scent. Patchouli also has a reputation as an aphrodisiac, a notion that probably originated in India, where it is used as an anointing oil in Tantric sexual practices. Perfumers must think that it works since minute quantities of high quality oil scent such famous perfumes as Tabu and Shocking. All attempts to make a synthetic patchouli have failed utterly.

PRINCIPAL CONSTITUENTS: Patchoulol (up to 50 percent), patchoulene (similar to azulene), pogostol, bulnesol, bulnese, eugenol, cadinene, carvone, and benzoic and cinnamic aldehydes, among others

SCENT: The odor is heavy, earthy, musty, pungent, and penetrating.

THERAPEUTIC PROPERTIES: Antidepressant, anti-inflammatory, antiseptic, antiviral, and antifungal; reduces fluid retention

USED FOR: Cosmetically, the essential oil is a cell rejuvenator and antiseptic that treats a number of skin problems, including eczema and inflamed, cracked, and mature skin. As an antifungal, it counters athlete's foot. The aroma reduces appetite and helps to relieve headaches, unless the patient doesn't like it! Add 8 drops per ounce to a hair conditioner to help eliminate dandruff.

Peppermint

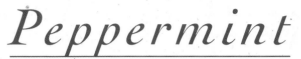

(Mentha piperita)

Family: Lamiaceae (Labiatae)

The most widely used of all aromatic oils, peppermint makes a grand and obvious appearance in all sorts of edible and nonedible products, including beverages, ice cream, sauces and jellies, liqueurs, medicines, dental preparations, cleaners, cosmetics, tobacco, desserts, and gums.

It was known to the Egyptians, who dedicated mint to the god Horus. The Romans personified it as *Minthe* or *Mentha*, the beautiful naiad loved by Pluto, god of the underworld. When Pluto's queen, Proserpine, saw what was going on she jealously trampled Minthe, transforming her into the lowly plant. But Pluto decreed that the more mint was walked on the sweeter it would smell.

Peppermint self-hybridized by the seventeenth century into more than 20 modern varieties of square-stemmed perennials that easily spread by underground root systems. It now grows wild throughout Europe, North America, and Australia, and is one of the few essential oil plants grown in the

U.S., where the rainfall, temperature, and soil conditions in Michigan and central Oregon are ideal for high oil production. Most of the oil is redistilled to produce a lighter mint flavor for candies and gums.

After the *British Medical Journal* noted in 1879 that smelling menthol, which is the main component in peppermint, relieves headaches and nerve pain, menthol cones that evaporate into the air became all the rage. Taking center stage in several controversies, herbalists have long argued for or against the assertion by the ancient Greek physician Galen that peppermint is an aphrodisiac. But everyone, including modern scientists, agrees that it is a strong mental and physical stimulant that can help one concentrate and stay awake and alert.

PRINCIPAL CONSTITUENTS: Menthol (up to 70 percent), menthone, menthyl acetate, limonene, pulegone, cineol, azulene, and others

SCENT: Peppermint has a powerful, minty-fresh, camphoraceous, cool, and distinctive fragrance.

THERAPEUTIC PROPERTIES: Anti-inflammatory; relieves pain, muscle spasms, and cramping; relaxes the nerves; kills viral infections; decreases gas and indigestion; clears lung congestion; reduces fever

USED FOR: Peppermint helps the digestion of heavy foods and relieves flatulence and intestinal cramping, actually relaxing the digestive muscles so they operate more efficiently. A massage over the abdomen with an oil containing peppermint can greatly aid intestinal spasms, indigestion, nausea, and irritable bowel syndrome. Peppermint essential oil is included in most liniments, where it warms by increasing blood flow, relieving muscle spasms and arthritis. Peppermint relieves the itching of ringworm, herpes simplex, scabies, and poison oak. It also clears sinus and lung congestion when inhaled directly or when a vapor balm is rubbed on the chest. It also destroys many bacteria and viruses. Peppermint is not drying, as one might assume; rather, it stimulates the skin's oil production, so use it blended with other oils to treat dry complexions. When using peppermint, remember that it is an energizing scent.

WARNINGS: Watch out! At first peppermint feels cooling, but too much of it can burn.

Rose

(Rosa damascena, R. gallica, and others)
Family: Rosaceae

The fragrance of rose has long inspired poets and lovers. One legend says the red rose came from the blood of the Greek love goddess Aphrodite. The name of Aphrodite's son Eros, god of love, is an anagram for rose. Folktales that come from China to Europe tell similar stories about the rose's symbolism as the unfolding of both spiritual and physical love and perfection.

Originally from Asia Minor, the plant was brought by Turkish merchants to Bulgaria, where the most valued oil is now produced. It is gentle and nontoxic but costly, because so little can be made during distillation and because the bushes need so much care. The oil is distilled or solvent-extracted from blossoms; but, as it is difficult to separate from water, the oil must be distilled at least twice, resulting in two products. The first is called attar of roses; the by-product is called rose water. The unadulterated oil congeals when it cools, but can be liquefied again by the warmth of the hand. It has been an age-old favorite essential oil in facial creams because, in addition to its incredible fragrance, it is reputed to fend off aging. It is also used in costly perfumes.

PRINCIPAL CONSTITUENTS: Geraniol (up to 75 percent), citronellol, nerol, stearopten, phenyl ethanol, farnesol, and others

SCENT: Wonderfully intense, the fragrance is sweet and floral.

THERAPEUTIC PROPERTIES: Antidepressant, antiseptic, anti-inflammatory, astringent, antibacterial, and antiviral; increases menstruation, calms nervous tension

USED FOR: A cell rejuvenator and powerful antiseptic, rose essential oil soothes and heals skin conditions, including cuts and burns. Rose treats asthma and can be used as an inhalant, albeit an expensive one. Instead, most people reserve it for skin creams and lotions; it is suitable for all complexion types. It helps a variety of female disorders, possibly by balancing hormones. A massage oil helps various types of female problems, including menstrual cramps, PMS symptoms, and moodiness during menopause. Many women report that simply smelling rose's fragrance is enough to do the trick. Sniffing the oil or using a massage oil containing rose has even been suggested to help reverse impotency.

Rosemary

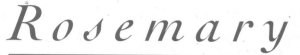

(Rosmarinus officinalis)
Family: Lamiaceae (Labiatae)

The ancients believed that rosemary strengthened memory, and thus it became an emblem of fidelity, important at both weddings and funerals. The smoke was inhaled to protect against brain weakness and dizziness, and the herb was burned in schools and universities to inspire the pupils. Japanese researchers have preliminary evidence that rosemary does indeed improve memory. Rosemary was burned by the poor instead of frankincense; the old French name for it, *incensier*, came from rosemary's celebrated history as church incense. Until the twentieth century, the fragrant branches were burned in French hospitals, with juniper, to purify the air. Rosemary also made its impression on early cosmetics; it was the main ingredient in the famous fourteenth century "Hungary Water," which is still available today. This Mediterranean native with tiny, pale blue flowers that bloom in late winter loves growing by the ocean — its name *rosmarinus* means "dew of the sea." It is cultivated worldwide, although France, Spain, and Tunisia are the main producers of the essential oil.

PRINCIPAL CONSTITUENTS: Borneol, camphene, camphors, cineol, verbenone, pinenes, limonene, linalol, terpineol, and others

SCENT: The odor is herbaceous, woody, sharp, and camphorous.

THERAPEUTIC PROPERTIES: Antiseptic, astringent, antioxidant; relieves rheumatic and muscle pain, relaxes nerves, improves digestion and appetite, increases sweating

USED FOR: As an ingredient in a massage oil, compress, or bath, rosemary essential oil is excellent for increasing poor circulation and easing muscle and rheumatism pain. It is especially penetrating when used in a liniment. It is very antiseptic, so inhaling the essential oil or adding it to a vapor balm that is rubbed on the chest and throat relieves lung congestion and sore throat. It is a stimulant to the nervous system and increases energy. Cosmetically it encourages dry, mature skin to produce more of its own natural oils. It also helps get rid of canker sores. Add it to shampoos—it is an age-old remedy for dandruff and hair loss.

WARNINGS: It can be overly stimulating and

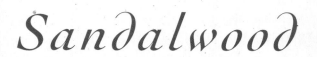

Sandalwood

(Santalum album)
Family: Santalaceae

Sandalwood is distilled from the roots and heartwood of trees that take 50 to 80 years to reach full maturity. In an amazing and lengthy manufacturing process used since ancient times, the mature sandalwood trees are cut down, then left to be eaten by ants, which consume all but the fragrant heartwood and roots. Every part of the heartwood is used, including the sawdust. The scent, called *chandana*, is used to induce a calm and meditative state. The lasting fragrance only improves with age. According to mythology, sandalwood originally grew only in heaven's gardens. Temple gates and religious statues are carved from the wood because of this spiritual association, the exquisite scent, and because it is impermeable to termites and other insects. Sandalwood also has an age-old reputation as an aphrodisiac, and in fact, its fragrance is similar to the human pheromone, *alpha androsterole*. Mysore, India, produces the finest quality oil, and as an endangered species, sandalwood is regulated by the Indian government, which now grows the trees in cultivated plantations.

PRINCIPAL CONSTITUENTS: Santalols (up to 90 percent), fusanol, santene, santalic acid, teresantol, borneol, santalone, and others

SCENT: It has a soft, warm, woody, and balsamic fragrance.

THERAPEUTIC PROPERTIES: Antidepressant, anti-inflammatory, antifungal, astringent, sedative, insecticide, urinary and lung antiseptic; relieves lung congestion and nausea

USED FOR: The essential oil treats infections of the reproductive organs, especially in men, and helps relieve bladder infections. For either use, add 12 drops of essential oil for every ounce of vegetable oil and use as a massage oil over the infected area. This oil also counters inflammation, so it can be used on hemorrhoids. A syrup or chest balm containing sandalwood helps relieve persistent coughs and sore throat. One of sandalwood's most important uses is to sedate the nervous system, subduing nervousness, anxiety, insomnia, and to some degree, reducing nerve pain. Researchers have found it relaxes brain waves. Suitable for all complexion types, it is especially useful on rashes, inflammation, acne, and dry, dehydrated, or chapped skin.

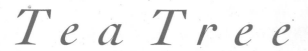

Tea Tree

(Melaleuca alternifolia)
Family: Myrtaceae

On his first voyage to Australia, Captain Cook made a sharp-tasting tea from tea tree leaves and later used them in brewing beer. Eventually the leaves and then the essential oil were used to purify water. Australian soldiers and sailors used the essential oil as an all-purpose healing agent during World War II.

It's only recently, however, that essential oil companies have begun touting tea tree's healing properties. Medical journal articles support reports of its ability to heal mouth infections, and its primary use is in products for gum infection and canker sores, germicidal soaps, and deodorants. You will find several variations of tea tree, such as the harsher cajeput (*M. cajuputii*) and niaouli (*M. viridiflora*), favored for treating viral infections such as herpes. There is also a tea tree oil that is simply called MQV (*M. quinquenervia viridiflora*). Although it is more expensive, some aromatherapists prefer its softer, sweeter fragrance.

PRINCIPAL CONSTITUENTS: Terpineol (as high as 30–40 percent), cineol, pinene, cymene, and others

SCENT: Astringent, acrid, camphorous, and medicinal, the scent is similar to eucalyptus. Poor quality oil smells like melted rubber.

THERAPEUTIC PROPERTIES: Anti-inflammatory, antiviral, antibacterial, antifungal; destroys parasitic infections, encourages the healing of wounds, clears lung and sinus congestion, stimulates immune system

USED FOR: Called a "medicine cabinet in a bottle," tea tree is effective against bacteria, fungi, and viruses and stimulates the immune system. Use it in compresses, salves, massage oil, and washes to fight all sorts of infections, including herpes, shingles, chicken pox, candida, thrush, flu, cold, and those of the urinary tract. Studies show that the presence of blood and pus from infection only increase tea tree's antiseptic powers. It heals wounds, protects skin from radiation burns from cancer therapy, and encourages scar tissue to regenerate. Tea tree also treats diaper rash, acne, wounds, and insect bites. Adding just one drop to dish and diaper washing rinses gets rid of bacteria. It is one of the most nonirritating antiseptic oils, but this varies with the species, so a few people do find it slightly irritating.

Thyme

(Thymus vulgaris)

Family: Lamiaceae (Labiatae)

Most people consider this low-growing perennial evergreen no more than a culinary seasoning, yet its fragrance led Rudyard Kipling to write of "our close-bit thyme that smells like dawn in paradise." Ancient Greeks so highly regarded its aroma that to compliment someone they would say the person smelled like thyme.

Thymain, a derivative of the name, described burning incense, and the "art of using perfumes as medicine" was known as *thymiatechny*. The word thyme also relates to strength, spirit, or courage—attributes thought to be imparted to anyone who sniffed its fragrant leaves. Medieval ladies sent a sprig of the herb with their knights to instill these virtues in them during travel and battle.

Thyme was used in Muslim countries for fumigating houses; frankincense was added when people could afford it. The compound thymol, derived from thyme essential oil, is one of the strongest antiseptics known and has been isolated as an ingredient in drugstore gargles, mouthwashes, cough drops, and vapor chest balms. Some of the best known products that contain thymol are Listerine mouthwash and Vicks VapoRub.

PRINCIPAL CONSTITUENTS: Thymol and carvacrol (highly antiseptic but potentially toxic), cymene, terpinene, camphene, borneol, linalol, menthone, geraniol, citral, thuyanol, and many more

SCENT: The scent is herbaceous, strong, hot, penetrating, and therapeutic.

THERAPEUTIC PROPERTIES: Antiseptic, antibacterial, antifungal, antioxidant, astringent; destroys parasitic infections, helps dissipate muscle and rheumatic pain, stops coughing, decreases gas and indigestion, stimulates menstruation, clears lung congestion, stimulates the immune system and circulation

USED FOR: Thyme essential oil is primarily used in a compress or sometimes in a salve or cream to fight serious infection. Stir 8 drops of the oil into a salve or cream or add them to a cup of water and soak a cloth in it to make a compress. It is also useful for treating gum and mouth infections, such as thrush (*Candida*). You can make your own mouthwash by adding three drops of thyme essential oil to ¼ ounce tincture of Oregon grape root and ¾ ounce water. Shake well before rinsing your mouth; then spit it out. You can relieve lung and sinus congestion and infection by adding a couple drops of thyme essential oil to a quart of simmering water and inhaling the steam, although the essential oils of eucalyptus, tea tree, or lavender are preferable for steaming because they are less toxic than thyme.

WARNINGS: Thyme essential oil can irritate the skin and mucus membranes as well as raise blood pressure, so be sure to use it only in very low dilutions. Red thyme oil is even stronger than the white and is rarely used, except in a liniment for its increased heating effects. Essential oils of thyme are sometimes available in which the most potent components, thymol and carvacrol, are removed, although this decreases their antiseptic properties. Thyme essential oil should not be used with pregnant women or children. Thyme does destroy intestinal worms, but the essential oil should never be taken internally. Instead, use the herb itself in the form of a tea or tincture.

Ylang Ylang

(Cananga odorata)

Family: Annonaceae

Originating in the Philippines, ylang ylang means "flower of flowers" or "fragrance of all fragrances." This fragrance is traditionally used to sharpen the senses and to temper depression, fear, anger, and jealousy. For these reasons, and also because of its reputation as an aphrodisiac, the flowers are spread on the beds of the newly married in Indonesia. Modern aromatherapists find the scent strongly sedating, easily sending the most reluctant sleeper off to dreamland. Science, on the other hand, regards ylang ylang more as a mental stimulant. Can it be both? Quite possibly it stimulates people's minds in one way while relaxing them in another. Ylang ylang is also widely used as a cosmetic when mixed with coconut oil. People throughout the tropics use it to protect their hair from salt water damage. Today, as one of the most abundant and least expensive of the true floral-smelling essential oils, it is a favorite in perfumes and cosmetics and is even added to some beverages and desserts. The essential oil varies greatly due to climatic and botanical differences. As a result, there are several commercial grades with distinct scents.

PRINCIPAL CONSTITUENTS: Linalol, geraniol, eugenol, safrol, ylangol, linalyl benzoate, linalyl acetate, alpha pinene, benzoic acid, cadinene, caryophylelene, creosol, isoeugenol

SCENT: The fragrance is intensely sweet, heady, floral, and slightly spicy, with a narcissus or bananalike overtone.

THERAPEUTIC PROPERTIES: Antidepressant; stimulates circulation, relieves muscle spasms, lowers blood pressure, relaxes nerves

USED FOR: Of all the essential oils, ylang ylang is one of the best at relaxing the mind and the body. Simply sniffing it can slightly lower blood pressure, although taking a bath with the oil or using it in a massage oil greatly enhances the relaxation experience. It can be helpful in cases of stress, shock, or anxiety. When used as a hair tonic, it balances oil production. Add about 6 drops to every ounce of hair conditioner.

WARNINGS: High concentrations of ylang ylang can produce headaches or nausea. Some people are more susceptible than others to this effect and will generally react immediately.

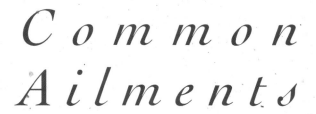

Common Ailments

The following simple aromatherapy treatments are for relatively minor problems that you would normally treat at home. The treatment recipes that follow were designed so that you can start making your own aromatherapy preparations after buying only a few essential oils. The proportions have been carefully chosen to make the product both very therapeutic and pleasant to smell. For an introduction to the rules of aromatherapy blending and lots of helpful tips, be sure to read "Getting Started" before you begin making any of these recipes.

Using the Remedies

Many remedies given in this chapter are used as a massage or bath oil. That's because the safest way to use essential oils is externally and in a diluted state. You should never ingest them. Massage techniques vary—some cover the whole body while others work on only a part of it. Acupressure is an example of a method that requires very little, if any, massage oil. Techniques such as Swedish massage and lymphatic massage call for repeated applications of massage oil. If you find yourself using a tablespoon of massage oil or more at one session, use half the amount of essential oils in the recipe. Remember, the best aromatherapy is achieved when the fragrance is subtle, not overpowering. Cut the amount of essential oils in half when the aromatherapy product will be used on the elderly, children younger than 12 years of age, or someone who is very ill or frail.

Good judgment and common sense are the most important ingredients to use when self-prescribing and treating. Sometimes ailments that seem relatively minor can actually be indications of far more troubling problems. It's a good idea to get professional advice whenever you are in doubt about what you have or how to treat it. Also, don't abandon your prescription drugs in favor of aromatherapy treatments unless you get professional advice that it will be safe to do so.

While aromatherapy offers gentle and effective forms of therapy, you will often get quicker and better results when you combine it with other natural treatments. In many cases, adding herbal remedies, lifestyle changes, and nutritional supplements to your aromatherapy regimen will help you to heal faster and better. In some cases, using the herbs from which the essential oils are made is safer than trying to properly dilute essential oils. This is particularly true when the herb is more effective when it is taken internally. Although you should not ingest essential oils, you can safely drink herb teas such as peppermint to settle your stomach or chamomile to relax you before bed.

Aromatherapy can be a valuable healing tool; however, not all illnesses can be treated with essential oils. Conditions such as diabetes, chronic kidney disease, and multiple sclerosis are not candidates for aromatherapy treatment because they require much more extensive therapy than offered by aromatic chemicals. You can, however, use aromatherapy to relieve many of the symptoms caused by the above disorders, such as the circulation problems that occur with diabetes and the water retention resulting from kidney disease. Aromatherapy is also an excellent way to help you deal with stress, which often compromises physical and emotional well-being and even triggers many seemingly unrelated disorders. Aromatherapy will also go a long way toward boosting your own ability to handle the overall problem by helping you handle the stress. The conditions listed in this book are a good guide to and indication of the kind of ailments best treated by aromatherapy.

Oils used in the treatment recipes can all be found in the profiles in the previous chapter.

GETTING CREATIVE

After you've tried your hand at making a few aromatherapy formulas, you'll probably get ideas about how to alter them to better fit your personal needs, make the fragrance more appealing, or make substitutions because you don't have an oil or two used in the recipe. Feel free to experiment and make your own concoctions.

• Each condition discussed contains a list of essential oils suitable for treating it. This is where you should start if you want to make alterations.

• Read about the oils you want to use in the Essential Oils chapter. The information will help you determine your best options based on their individual characteristics.

• "Getting Started," on the practice of aromatherapy, will give you some ideas about the relative strengths of oils in a blend and proportions to use, as well as many ways to use them.

Helpful Hints Before You Begin

• In recipes that call for 12 drops of an essential oil, you might prefer using the equivalent measurement of $\frac{1}{8}$ teaspoon.

• In recipes that require vegetable oil, any will do. However, almond or canola oils are preferred by most people because they are easy to obtain and don't have their own scent. A wide variety of other oils are available at natural food stores—feel free to experiment.

• If you plan to keep a preparation longer than six months, use the more expensive jojoba oil rather than vegetable oil because it won't ever go rancid. Or add one or two capsules of vitamin E, which will preserve your recipe longer than other oils, but not as long as jojoba.

• When preparing recipes to be used by the elderly, the very young (less than 12 years of age), or anyone who is very ill or frail, be sure to cut the amount of essential oils in half, keeping the carrier (vegetable oil, water, alcohol, vinegar, etc.) the same. These people are so sensitive that they will react equally well to the smaller amount.

• Just want to try something out? Make a smaller amount by cutting the proportions in half. If the drops don't divide evenly, use the smaller number. Use a clean toothpick if you only want a smidgen of something, such as patchouli (yes, it's that powerful!).

Acne and Oily Skin

Acne may not be a hazard to your health, but it does impair your looks. The problem typically is the result of clogged skin pores. When the pores and follicles (canals that contain hair shafts) are blocked, oil cannot be secreted and builds up. Bacteria feeds on the oil and multiplies. People with oily skin have a greater chance of developing acne, as do teenagers and anyone experiencing hormonal fluctuations. Although not medically proven, stress may also contribute to acne breakouts.

Luckily, quite an array of essential oils are available to help you deal with acne. That's because many oils help manage the specific underlying problems that cause acne: They balance hormones, reduce stress, improve the complexion, and regulate the skin's oil production. This makes aromatherapy the ideal treatment for blemishes, pimples, and other skin eruptions. Commercial acne remedies have long recognized this. Noxema, for example, relies on eucalyptus essential oil as its primary active ingredient because it reduces oil production and fights bacterial infection at the same time.

A salt and essential oil compress (see Zit Zap Compress recipe, page 172) is a good way to start your acne home care program. For persistent or especially troublesome eruptions, immediately follow the compress with the Intensive Blemish Treatment on page 172.

If you have oily skin, use the facial toner below daily. Or you can choose from any of the skin-drying and antiseptic essential oils from the following list, and then dilute them in a base of witch hazel and aloe vera gel, both of which are readily available at drugstores. The witch hazel contains alcohol, so it is especially drying, and there's no disputing that aloe vera is one of the most beneficial and healing herbs to put on your skin. Combine these with essential oils and prepare yourself for a dazzling complexion!

Essential oils for acne or an oily complexion: cedarwood, clary sage, eucalyptus, frankincense, geranium, juniper berry, lavender, lemon, lemongrass, sandalwood, tea tree

FACIAL TONER FOR OILY COMPLEXIONS

12 drops lemongrass oil
6 drops juniper berry oil
2 drops ylang ylang oil
1 ounce witch hazel lotion
1 ounce aloe vera gel

Combine all of the ingredients in a glass bottle. Give the mixture a good shake and it's done! Apply at least once a day. If you find witch hazel too drying, vinegar is an excellent substitute. It is not as drying as the witch hazel lotion and helps to retain the skin's natural acid balance.

ZIT ZAP COMPRESS

4 drops cedarwood oil
2 drops eucalyptus oil
1 teaspoon Epsom salts
¼ cup water

Pour the boiling water over the Epsom salts.
When the salts are dissolved and the water has
cooled just enough to not burn the skin, add
the essential oils. Soak a small absorbent cloth
in the hot solution, then press the cloth against
the blemishes for about one minute. Repeat
several times by rewetting the cloth in the
same solution.

INTENSIVE BLEMISH TREATMENT

12 drops tea tree oil
½ teaspoon Oregon grape root, powdered
a few drops of water
800 units vitamin E (optional)

Stir the water and essential oil into the herb
powder to make a paste. Apply as a mask
directly on the blemished area. Let the paste
dry and keep it on your skin for at least
20 minutes, then rinse off. This routine can be
done more than once a day, if you wish. The
vitamin E can be obtained by poking open a
vitamin capsule and squeezing out the oil. It is
a good addition when obstinate sores need to
heal or if there is any chance of scarring.

Asthma

The characteristic wheezing of asthma is made by the effort to push air through swollen, narrowed bronchial passages. During an asthma attack, stale air cannot be fully exhaled because the bronchioles are swollen and clogged with mucous, and thus less fresh air can be inhaled. The person gasps and labors for breath. Allergic reactions to food, stress, and airborne allergens are the common causes of asthma. Allergies trigger production of histamine, which dilates blood vessels and constricts airways. Asthma sufferers fight an ongoing battle with such low-level congestion, which is actually an attempt by unhappy lungs to rid themselves of irritations.

Many aromatherapy books warn against using essential oils to treat asthma. Some asthmatics are sensitive to fragrance and find that it triggers their attacks. While you certainly don't want to make the situation any worse, aromatherapy offers promising results when used judiciously.

The safest time for aromatherapy treatments is in between attacks. Use a chest rub made from essential oils that have decongestive and antihistamine properties, such as peppermint and ginger. German chamomile, which contains chamazulene, is thought to actually prevent the release of histamine. Frankincense, marjoram, and rose encourage deep breathing and allow lungs to expand. To reduce bronchial spasms, use the relaxants: chamomile, lavender, rose, geranium, and marjoram.

A lavender steam can be used by some asthmatics even during an attack. The steam opens airways, while lavender quickly relaxes lung spasms. This may halt the attack right in its tracks or at least make it less severe. As an added bonus, lavender also relaxes the mind, so it helps dissipate the panic you feel when you can't catch your breath. Follow the instructions for steam-

ASTHMA INHALATION RUB

6 drops lavender oil
4 drops geranium oil
1 drop marjoram oil
1 drop peppermint or ginger oil
1 ounce vegetable oil

Combine the ingredients. Rub on chest as needed, especially before bedtime. Since asthmatics can be extremely sensitive to scent, do a sniff test first. Test the formula by simply sniffing it to make sure there is no adverse reaction.

ing under Congestion, Sinus and Lung on pages, 179–180. If you find that steaming only makes it more difficult to breathe, use an aromatherapy diffuser or a humidifier instead. For babies and small children, put some very hot water in the bathtub, add several drops of lavender essential oil, and hold the child in your arms over the steam. You can also rub someone's feet with an aromatherapy massage oil.

Essential oils are not powerful enough to heal an asthmatic condition all by themselves. Herbs that repair lung damage and improve breathing are also needed, along with avoiding whatever sparks the allergic reaction. If this means stress, then other aromatherapy techniques such as massage, relaxation techniques, and fragrant baths can help you de-stress your life.

Essential oils for asthma: chamomile, eucalyptus (don't use during an attack), frankincense (deepens breathing, allows lungs to expand), geranium, ginger, lavender, marjoram, peppermint, rose

Bladder Infection

Bladder infections are common, especially in women. So common, in fact, that you may already be familiar with the medical term cystitis to describe the inflammation that can result when bladder infections are unattended. Fortunately, several essential oils can come to the rescue. Juniper berry, sandalwood, chamomile, pine, tea tree, and bergamot are especially effective treatments. However, juniper berry is so strong that it could irritate the kidneys if the bladder infection has spread into them. If that is the case, stick to the other oils. In fact, if there is any chance that you have a kidney infection, be sure to seek a doctor's opinion, as it can have serious consequences.

Apply a massage oil or a compress containing the essential oils listed in the recipe over the bladder, which is located under the lower abdomen, once or twice daily as an adjunct to herbal, nutritional, or even drug treatments.

Added to a bath, these same essential oils can be used during an active infection and will help prevent future infections. If taking a full bath isn't practical, then try a sitz bath. As the name implies, you simply sit in a large tub of warm water (see Uterine Problems, pages 234–237, for more information about using sitz baths).

Essential oils for bladder infections: bergamot, cedarwood, cypress, fir, frankincense, juniper berry (don't use if there's a kidney infection), sandalwood, tea tree

BLADDER INFECTION OIL

8 drops juniper berry or cypress oil
6 drops tea tree oil
6 drops bergamot oil
2 drops fennel oil
2 ounces vegetable oil

Combine the ingredients. Massage over the bladder area once daily. For a preventive treatment, add a tablespoon of this same oil to your bath.

Burns and Sunburn

The first step in treating any minor burn or sunburn is to quickly immerse the afflicted area in cold water (about 50°F) containing a few drops of essential oil. Or you can apply a cold compress that has been soaked in the same water. If the person feels overheated or if the eyelids are sunburned, place the compress on the forehead.

Burned skin is tender to the touch, so spraying a remedy is preferable to dabbing it on. A spray also is extra cooling and is especially handy when sunburn covers a large area.

For your burn wash, compress, or spray, lavender is an all-time favorite among aromatherapists. Lavender and aloe vera juice both promote new cell growth, reduce inflammation, stop infection, and decrease pain. Aloe has even been used successfully on radiation burns. There are several other essential oils that reduce the pain of burns and help them heal, so feel free to experiment. Use them in the same proportions suggested for lavender, except rose oil for which 1 drop equals 5 drops of other essential oils.

A small amount of vinegar helps to heal a minor burn and provides an additional cooling effect, but it is painful on an open wound. Reserve it for cases in which the skin is unbroken. In general, stick to treating minor, first-degree burns at home, and leave the care of deeper or more extensive burns to a doctor.

Essential oils for burns and sunburn: chamomile, geranium, lavender, marjoram, peppermint (cooling in small amounts), rose, tea tree

EMERGENCY BURN WASH/COMPRESS

5 drops lavender oil
1 pint water, about 50°F

Add the essential oil to the water and stir well to disperse the oil. Immerse the burned area for several minutes, or take a soft cloth, soak it in the water, and apply it to the burn. Leave the compress on for several minutes, then resoak and reapply at least twice more.

SUNBURN SOOTHER

20 drops lavender oil
4 ounces aloe vera juice
200 IU vitamin E oil
1 tablespoon vinegar

Combine ingredients. Shake well before using. Keep this remedy in a spritzer bottle, and use as often as needed. If you keep the spray in the refrigerator, the coolness will provide extra relief. For the best healing, make sure you use aloe vera juice and not drugstore gel. Apply as often as possible until you are healed.

Congestion, Sinus and Lung

The most common cause of sinus and lung congestion is a cold or flu virus. Additionally, secondary bacterial infections-that follow on the heels of colds and flus can be especially nasty, irritating the delicate lining in the respiratory tract. The mucous that causes the congestion is produced to protect that lining and wash away the infection.

For quick relief, thin out congestion by using the essential oils of eucalyptus, peppermint, and bergamot combined with steam. Remember how much easier it is to breath when you step into a steamy, hot shower? The steam opens up tightened bronchial passages, allowing the essential oils to penetrate and wipe out the viral or bacterial infection that is causing the problem.

Two of the best essential oils to eliminate infection are lavender and eucalyptus. In fact, studies prove that a two percent dilution of eucalyptus oil kills 70 percent of airborne staphylococcus bacteria. Anise, peppermint, and eucalyptus reduce coughing, perhaps by suppressing the brain's cough reflex. If congestion is severe, also use essential oils that loosen congestion, such as those listed on page 186. Cypress dries a persistently runny nose.

To create a therapeutic steam, add a few drops of essential oil to a pan of water that is simmering on the stove. You can also use a humidifier — some actually provide a compartment for essential oils. If you are at the office or traveling and steaming is impractical, try inhaling a tissue scented with the oils, or use a natural nasal inhaler. These are available in natural food and drugstores, or you can make your own using the recipe opposite. If you don't have a diffuser but would like to disinfect the air, simply combine water and essential oils and dispense the solution from a spray bottle.

A vapor balm (a salve containing essential oils) or massage oil can be rubbed over the chest, back, and throat to relieve congestion. Vapor balms increase circulation and warmth in the chest as they are absorbed through the skin. Placing a flannel cloth on the chest after rubbing in the oil will increase the warming action. Commercial products, such as Vicks VapoRub, still use derivatives of essential oils (or their synthetic oil counterparts) such as thymol from thyme and menthol from mint, in a petroleum ointment base, but more natural alternatives are available from your natural food store. Essential oil molecules are also easily inhaled from the balm.

The steam recipe given here uses eucalyptus, which is simple and effective, but you can replace it with any of the essential oils listed except clove and thyme, which can be too harsh when inhaled. However, all the oils given can be used in a vapor balm. If you are having trouble deciding which oils to use, refer to the essential oil profiles to determine their differences and which oil might have additional qualities that you would like to include.

Essential oils for fighting respiratory infections: benzoin, clove, eucalyptus, lavender, marjoram, tea tree, thyme

Essential oils to ease mucous congestion: benzoin, birch, cedarwood, clove, cypress, eucalyptus, ginger, peppermint, tea tree, thyme

NASAL INHALER

5 drops eucalyptus oil
¼ teaspoon coarse salt

Place the salt in a small vial (glass is best) with a tight lid and add essential oil. The salt will absorb the oil so it won't spill when you carry it. When needed, open the vial and inhale deeply. This same technique can be used with any essential oil listed above. Sniff as needed throughout the day.

VAPOR RUB

12 drops eucalyptus oil
5 drops peppermint oil
5 drops thyme oil
1 ounce olive oil

Combine ingredients in a glass bottle. Shake well to mix oils evenly. Gently massage into chest and throat. Use one to five times per day and especially just before bed.

Essential Oil Steam

¼ teaspoon eucalyptus oil
3 cups of water

Bring water to a simmer, turn off heat, and add essential oils. Set the pan where you can sit down next to it. Place your face over the steam and drape a towel over the back of your head to form a mini-sauna. Breathe in the steam, coming out for fresh air as needed. Do at least three rounds of steam inhalation several times a day. Fresh or dried eucalyptus leaves can be added to the water instead of the pure essential oil. You can replace the eucalyptus oil with other essential oils listed, except bay, clove, or thyme. Whichever essential oil you use, be sure to keep your eyes closed while steaming. It's okay to use this steam as often as you like.

Cuts, Scrapes, and Bruises

Simple cuts and scrapes can easily be treated with antiseptic essential oils. A mist of diluted oil is an excellent way to apply them. Herbal salves containing antiseptic essential oils are also effective in treating scrapes or wounds that aren't too deep. See page 186 for instructions for adding oils to a premade salve. Need to protect your cut? Many of the resins and balsams such as benzoin, frankincense, and myrrh actually form a protective barrier over the wound that acts as an antiseptic "Band-Aid." In an emergency, don't forget that you can dab a little lavender or tea tree oil directly on a scrape as they are among the least irritating of oils.

Essential oils for cuts and scrapes: benzoin, eucalyptus, frankincense, geranium, lavender, lemon, myrrh, rose, tea tree

---

GERM FIGHTER SPRAY

12 drops tea tree oil
6 drops eucalyptus oil
6 drops lemon oil
2 ounces distilled water or herbal tincture

Combine the ingredients, and shake well to disperse the oils before each use. Dispense this formula from a spray bottle as needed on minor cuts, burns, or abrasions to prevent infection and speed healing. As an alternative to the distilled water, you can use a tincture made from an antiseptic herb such as Oregon grape root. If you do this, keep in mind that tinctures contain alcohol, which will make the essential oils disperse better and increase the antiseptic properties of the spray, but it will also sting more on an open wound. Apply immediately and then several times a day to keep the wound clean and encourage healing.

Depression/Anxiety

It's no secret that fragrance lifts and enhances one's mood. The aroma of many plants, such as the elegant orange blossom aroma of neroli or the closely related and less expensive petitgrain, as well as jasmine, sandalwood, and ylang ylang, relieve depression and anxiety. Modern aromatherapists agree with the seventeenth-century herbalist John Gerard, who recommended the use of clary sage to ease depression, paranoia, mental fatigue, and nervous disorders. Researchers at International Flavors and Fragrances, Inc., in New Jersey have found that orange reduces anxiety. East Indians traditionally use basil to prevent agitation and nightmares.

Fragrances are generally effective for people who have mild forms of depression that do not require drugs. And they can be especially helpful when the doctor is trying to wean patients off drugs. Aromatherapy can be used safely in conjunction with antidepressant medications because it will not interfere with the dosage or effect. If you are currently taking prescription drugs to deal with depression or anxiety, however, don't abruptly stop taking them or replace them with essential oils without your doctor's okay.

Massage and bath oils are probably the most relaxing forms of antidepressant aromatherapy. If you wish to make your environment more uplifting at home or at work, try using an aromatherapy room spray, or put the essential oils in an aromatherapy diffuser, potpourri cooker, or a pan of simmering water. You can make a constant companion of your favorite oil, or of a blend of oils from the following list, by carrying them in a small vial (see the instructions for making a nasal inhaler on page 181). Then, when you need a lift, just take a whiff.

Essential oils for relieving anxiety and depression: bergamot, cedarwood, cinnamon, clary sage, cypress, geranium, jasmine, lavender, lemon, marjoram, neroli, orange, sandalwood, rose, ylang ylang

UPLIFTING FORMULA

6 drops bergamot oil
3 drops petitgrain oil
3 drops geranium oil
1 drop neroli (expensive, so optional)
2 ounces vegetable oil

Combine all the ingredients. Use as a massage oil, add 1 or 2 teaspoons to your bath, or add 1 teaspoon to a foot bath. For an equally uplifting room or facial spritzer, substitute the same amount of water for the vegetable oil in this formula. Put the water formula in a spray bottle, and spritz or sniff throughout the day as needed.

Dermatitis, Psoriasis, and Eczema

Dermatitis is an inflammation of the skin that causes itching, redness, and skin lesions. It's difficult even for dermatologists to uncover the source of this bothersome skin problem. Some obvious causes, though, are contact with an irritant such as poison oak or ivy, harsh chemicals, or anything to which one is allergic. Stress also seems to be a contributing factor in many types of dermatitis. Essential oils that counter stress, soothe inflammation and itching, soften roughness, and are both antiseptic and drying are used to treat these skin conditions.

One type of dermatitis is eczema, a word that describes a series of symptoms rather than a disease. Eczema is characterized by crusty, oozing skin that itches and may feel like it burns. Psoriasis is a dermatitis with red lesions covered by silverlike scales that flake off. This condition can be hereditary, but its cause is unknown. It has an annoying tendency to come and go for no apparent reason.

One of the best vehicles for essential oils in these cases is an herbal salve that already contains a base of skin healing herbs such as comfrey and calendula. You can use a store-bought herbal salve or one that you make yourself. Stir in 15 drops (or less) of essential oils per ounce of salve. Since salves come in a two-ounce jar, that means adding no more than 30 drops; use less if the salve already contains some essential oils.

Secondary skin infections, which often occur with eczema, need to be treated with antiseptic essential oils, such as those suggested for acne.

Essential oils for dermatitis: birch, chamomile, lavender, peppermint (for itching), rosemary, tea tree

DERMATITIS SKIN CARE

8 drops tea tree oil
8 drops chamomile oil
1 teaspoon Oregon grape tincture
2 ounces healing salve

With a toothpick, stir the tincture and essential oils into the salve. This will make the salve semi-liquid. You can purchase the tincture at a natural food store. Apply one to four times a day.

Diaper Rash

Aromatherapy baby oil and powder can help protect your little one from diaper rash. The oil repels moisture, and the powder absorbs moisture and prevents chafing. Use one or the other with every diaper change, or more often if needed. Baby oil is also good for the skin. Make your own baby powder from plain old corn starch and essential oils.

Essential oils for diaper rash: chamomile, lavender, sandalwood, tea tree

AROMATHERAPY BABY OIL

6 drops lavender oil
2 drops chamomile oil
2 ounces vegetable oil

Combine the ingredients. Use after each
diaper change and as an all-over massage oil.
The same amount of lavender and chamomile
can also be stirred into a basic herbal salve
with a toothpick and used on the diaper area.

FRAGRANT BABY POWDER

20 drops (¼ teaspoon) lavender oil
5 drops mandarin or tangerine oil
½ pound corn starch

Put the corn starch in a plastic zip-lock bag
and drop in the essential oils. Tightly close the
bag, and toss back and forth to distribute the
oil, breaking up any clumps by pressing them
with your fingers through the bag. Let stand at
least four days to distribute the essential oil.
Spice, salt, or Parmesan cheese shakers with
large holes in their lids make good powder
applicators. Powder after each diaper
change or bath.

Dry Skin

A dry skin condition can mean rough, cracked hands and a flaky complexion that could eventually lead to excessive wrinkling. Skin conditions like psoriasis and eczema often go hand in hand with dry skin.

For any dry skin product, choose essential oils that balance the production of oil on the skin and also are anti-inflammatory so that they'll reduce irritation and its characteristic puffiness. If your dry skin is also mature skin, the historic "anti-aging" essential oils lavender, geranium, neroli, rosemary, and rose are particularly suitable. These essential oils are also thought to rejuvenate skin by encouraging new cell growth. Other excellent oils to use on dry skin are frankincense, myrrh, and sandalwood. Perhaps their skin rejuvenating characteristics are the reason they have been so highly valued over the last two thousand years!

In small amounts, peppermint increases the production of oil in the skin. Chamomile, carrot seed, and helichrysum reduce inflammation that can accompany dry skin conditions. The latter two even help get rid of precancerous skin conditions that usually appear as raised discolorations on areas most exposed to the sun, such as the hands and face.

The best way to treat dry skin is with essential oils added to a cream or lotion. Both of these contain water, not just oil as in salves and ointments. The water is absorbed by the skin to help resolve the dryness. Meanwhile, the oil in these products acts as a protective barrier to keep moisture from evaporating out of the skin. Try to purchase as pure a cream as possible. Your most likely bet is at a natural food store that sells cosmetics. You may even be able to find a cream that already contains essential oils that are good for your dry complexion. If not, purchase an unscented cream, and stir the oils into it yourself. One more thing that you can do for dry skin is to avoid soap, except when your face is honestly dirty. Instead, a gentle oatmeal scrub (see the recipe opposite) combined with essential oils should be sufficient.

Essential oils to prevent aging: geranium, lavender, neroli, rose, rosemary

Essential oils for dry skin: all the above oils and frankincense, myrrh, sandalwood

Essential oil to moisturize skin: peppermint

Essential oils for reducing inflammation and puffiness: chamomile, lavender

---

ANTI-AGING COMPLEXION CREAM

15 drops geranium oil
3 drops rose oil
2 drops frankincense or neroli oil
2 ounces complexion cream

Stir the essential oils into the cream. Use daily.

DRY COMPLEXION SCRUB

6 drops lavender oil
2 drops peppermint oil
1 tablespoon dried elder flowers, lavender, or
chamomile (optional)
2 tablespoons oatmeal
1 tablespoon cornmeal

Grind dry ingredients in a blender or electric coffee grinder. (Drugstores sell colloidal oatmeal, which needs no grinding.) Add the essential oils, and stir to distribute. Store in a closed container, and use instead of soap for cleansing your face. For clean skin, moisten 1 teaspoon with enough water to make a paste, dampen your face with a little water, then gently apply scrub. Rinse with warm water. Use this daily instead of soap.

Earache

An earache is most likely due to an infection. While this is not the sort of condition to treat exclusively with aromatherapy, an aromatherapy massage oil rubbed on the outside of the ear is an excellent adjunct to other treatments. Dilute an antiseptic essential oil like lavender or tea tree in olive oil. Lavender has the added benefit of helping to reduce inflammation. Gently rub this around the outside of the ear and down along the lymph nodes on the side of the neck.

Do not put it in the ear itself. Instead, make a warm compress using these same oils and place it directly over the ear. Always treat both ears, even if only one hurts, and continue treating them for a couple days after the pain is gone.

Essential oils for earache: lavender, tea tree

AROMATHERAPY EAR RUB

3 drops lavender oil
3 drops tea tree oil
1 tablespoon vegetable oil

Combine ingredients. Rub this oil around the ear and down the side of the neck. For children, remember to use half this dilution (no more than 3 drops total of essential oil to 1 tablespoon carrier oil). Rub on two to four times a day, especially before bed.

Eyestrain/ Inflammation

Eye strain is common in this day of computers and sight-intensive desk jobs. Of course, essential oils should never go directly into the eye, even when diluted. However, you can ease eye discomfort with either a cold or warm compress. For most eye problems such as sties or inflammation, use essential oils such as lavender or chamomile because they will reduce the swelling.

Follow the suggestions for making a compress for headaches on page 200. For eyestrain, use a warm compress. To reduce inflammation, including that early morning eye puffiness, try using a cold compress. If you have the time, relax with the compress on your eyes for at least five minutes, although even a couple of minutes will provide some benefit.

A quick treatment for eyestrain that is especially handy when traveling is to use chamomile tea bags. Since the smell of chamomile is soothing and relaxing, too, you will receive an additional aromatherapy treatment to relieve the stress of the road.

Essential oils for eyestrain and inflammation: chamomile, lavender

EYE TEA

2 bags of chamomile tea

Steep the tea bags for a few minutes in a couple tablespoons of hot water, as if making a very strong tea. Let cool just enough so that it is comfortable for a warm treatment or cool at least to room temperature for a cool treatment. Lie down and place a tea bag over each eye, then cover with a soft cloth. Use as often as you like.

Fatigue

Just as some aromas calm you down, others will perk you up. Researchers found that this is especially true of eucalyptus and pine. The spicy aromas of clove, basil, black pepper, and cinnamon—and to a lesser degree patchouli,

---

PICK-ME-UP COMBO

8 drops lemon oil
2 drops eucalyptus oil
2 drops peppermint oil
1 drop cinnamon leaf oil
1 drop cardamom oil (expensive, so optional)
2 ounces vegetable oil

Combine the ingredients. Use as a massage oil, add 2 teaspoons to your bath, or add 1 teaspoon to a footbath. Without the vegetable oil, this combination can be used in an aromatherapy diffuser, simmering pan of water, or a potpourri cooker, or it can be added to 2 ounces of water for an air spray. The cardamom oil is optional, but, oh, does it enhance this massage oil! Use it as often as you like.

---

lemongrass, and sage—are other aromatherapy stimulants that reduce drowsiness, irritability, and headaches. Several large Tokyo companies circulate lemon, cypress, and peppermint through their air-conditioning and heating systems to keep employees alert. These stimulating essential oils have been shown to prevent the sharp drop in attention that typically hits after working for thirty minutes. Clove, cinnamon, lemon, cardamom, fennel, and angelica act as stimulants. Using aromatherapy stimulants is healthier for you than ingesting stimulants such as coffee because the scents provide energy without causing an adrenaline rush that strains the adrenal glands.

Essential oils for energy: cinnamon, clove, cypress, eucalyptus, fir, ginger, lemon, lemongrass, peppermint, rosemary

Fungal Infection/ Athlete's Foot

Many different fungal infections appear on the skin, and the following treatments can often wipe them out. Most people are familiar with ringworm, especially athlete's foot because it is so common. Athlete's foot is so common because feet sweat and then are cloistered in socks and shoes. This creates the moist environment that fungi really love. If sweating feet are part of the problem, you can use sage to decrease perspiration. Peppermint will help relieve the itching that accompanies a fungal infection. Incorporating the essential oils into a cornstarch powder or a vinegar-based preparation will discourage fungal growth because both are quite drying. Vinegar has the extra benefit of destroying fungal infections.

Some of the most effective antifungal essential oils are tea tree and eucalyptus; lemon eucalyptus is particularly helpful. Lavender, myrrh, and geranium are close seconds. A small amount of peppermint essential oil relieves the itching, and since it stimulates blood circulation, it helps perk you up after a long day on your feet. Don't hesitate to use the same essential oils to treat funguses that creep under nails or affect other parts of the body.

Aromatic Foot Bath

6 drops tea tree oil
4 drops sage oil
2 drops peppermint oil
1–2 quarts water
¼ cup Epsom salts (optional)

Fill a container that is big enough for both feet with very warm water. Add the essential oils, and soak your feet for at least 15 minutes. The Epsom salts are a good addition if your feet are sore or just plain "dog tired"! When making any type of foot bath, you can also add a drop of your own choice of essential oil for whatever emotional impact you need. For example, the peppermint suggested in this recipe is an emotional and physical pick-me-up. It feels great at the end of the day, every day, or at least twice a week.

FUNGAL FIGHTER SOLUTION

12 drops tea tree oil
8 drops geranium oil
3 drops thyme oil
2 drops myrrh oil (expensive, so optional)
1 tablespoon tincture of benzoin
2 ounces apple cider vinegar

Combine the ingredients, and shake well before each use. Dab this solution on the afflicted area, or use it as a wash at least once a day—more often if possible. You can purchase tincture of benzoin at any drugstore.

An aromatic foot bath is a great way to treat fungal conditions like athlete's foot or to simply revitalize feet after a long day. You simply can't ask for a better way to take your medicine! If you think you don't have time for such a luxury, why not haul the basin in front of the TV, or read the newspaper or a book while enjoying your soak. Get yourself a basin large enough to accommodate both feet, fill it with warm water, and add several drops of essential oil. Add Epsom salts to relax tight muscles and soreness.

For a complete anti-fungal treatment, start off with a foot bath, hand soak, or wash that covers the afflicted area. Afterward, dry off thoroughly, then apply the Fungal Fighter Solution with vinegar followed by the Fungal Fighter Powder.

Do the entire routine at least once a day, and apply either the vinegar or the powder a few extra times.

Essential oils for fungal infection: benzoin, clove, eucalyptus (especially lemon eucalyptus), geranium, lavender, lemongrass, myrrh, peppermint, sandalwood, tea tree, thyme

FUNGAL FIGHTER POWDER

14 drops lemon eucalyptus or tea tree oil
8 drops geranium oil
5 drops sage oil
1 drop peppermint oil
¼ cup cornstarch

Place the cornstarch in a resealable plastic bag. Sprinkle in the essential oils slowly, trying to distribute them evenly through the powder. Close the bag and toss the powder, breaking up any clumps that form. For long-term storage, keep the powder in a sealed plastic bag or glass or ceramic container, although you probably will find a shake bottle with a perforated lid more convenient to dispense it.

A variety of these are sold in housewares departments for the kitchen. Use at least once a day, more often if possible.

Headaches

Aromatherapy really proves its worth with headaches. Peppermint, eucalyptus, and lavender are especially helpful in reducing headache pain. A tincture of lavender called "Palsy Drops" was recognized by the *British Pharmacopoeia* for more than 200 years and used by physicians to relieve muscle spasms, nervousness, and headaches until the 1940s, when herbs and aroma preparations fell out of favor and chemicals became more popular. In a 1994 U.S. study by H. Gobel, the essential oils of peppermint and eucalyptus relaxed both the mind and muscles of headache sufferers when the oils were diluted in alcohol and rubbed on their foreheads. Essential oils can be also used to make a compress to place on your forehead whenever a headache hits.

Most people find that their headaches respond best to a cold compress, but you can use a warm or hot compress—or alternate the two—for the result that works best. You can also place a second compress at the back of the neck. When you do not have time for compresses, dab a small drop of lavender, eucalyptus, or peppermint oil on each temple. For some people, a hot bath only makes their head pound more. However, if bathing does ease your pain, add a few drops of relaxing lavender or chamomile to your bath water.

Migraine headaches can be especially painful. Raising the temperature of the hands 15°F by soaking them in warm water seems to short-circuit a vascular headache such as a migraine by regulating circulation. Adding a couple drops of

HEADACHE-BE-GONE COMPRESS

5 drops lavender or eucalyptus oil
1 cup cold water

Add essential oil to water, and swish a soft cloth in it. Wring out the cloth, lie down, and close your eyes. Place the cloth over your forehead and eyes. Use throughout the day, as often as you can.

MIGRAINE HEADACHE HAND SOAK

5 drops lavender oil
5 drops ginger oil
1 quart hot water, about 110°F

Add essential oils to the hot water, and soak hands for at least 3 minutes. This therapy can be done repeatedly.

essential oil to the water increases the effect. Migraines often respond best to a blend of ginger and lavender.

Cluster headaches can also be quite severe and require special treatment. In addition to the headache compress, try a cream made from capsaicin, the active compound in cayenne peppers.

RESTFUL HEADACHE PILLOW

12 drops lavender oil
12 drops marjoram oil
1 cup flax seeds
8½" × 9" piece of silk cloth

Add essential oils to flax seeds (found at any natural food store) in a glass jar and let them sit for a week until the oils are absorbed. Fold and stitch the cloth (an old scarf works fine) into a bag measuring approximately 4"×8½," and add the scented flax seeds. Sew up the opening. Lie down, and lay this "pillow" over your eyes when you feel a headache coming on. Store the pillow in a glass jar to preserve the scent. If the scent starts to dissipate, you can add more essential oil directly through the silk as needed.

Spread it on your forehead, temples, or any other area where you experience pain, but not too close to the eyes. Capsaicin blocks a neurotransmitter called substance P (which stands for pain), stopping pain impulses from registering in the brain. The cream works best as a preventative, keeping the headache from forming in the first place. Available for sale in drug and natural food stores, it needs to be applied four to five times a day for about four weeks to do much good, yet it is well worth-the trouble.

Essential oils for headaches: chamomile, cinnamon, clove, eucalyptus, ginger, jasmine, lavender, lemongrass, marjoram, patchouli, peppermint

Herpes

Herpes is a painful viral infection that appears on the genitals or around the mouth in the form of fever blisters. The herpes virus can lay dormant in the nervous system, appearing only now and then. Current conventional medicine has little to offer to treat herpes and does not know how to eliminate the virus. The virus reactivates when the immune system is weakened, such as when you are under emotional or physical stress. Consider using aromatherapy and other methods to build up your immune system and to relax.

Research shows that creams made from capsaicin, a compound found in cayenne, deadens the pain of herpes and shingles. Capsaicin creams are sold in drugstores and many natural food stores. The essential oils of cayenne will work if added to a cream or oil base, but go easy with it since too much can burn the skin. Small amounts of peppermint sometimes also diminish the nerve-tingling pain of herpes and shingles.

Tea tree, especially the type known as niaouli, is the favorite essential oil to treat herpes. Although much more expensive, an essential oil of myrrh is also very effective. Dilute the essential oil of your choice in an equal amount of vegetable oil or alcohol, and apply it directly to the herpes blisters. If applied as soon as the blisters begin to appear, any of these oils may prevent it from breaking out. This formula can be used on another virus related to herpes, called herpes zoster, which causes chicken pox and shingles.

Essential oils for herpes and shingles: bergamot, eucalyptus, geranium, myrrh, peppermint (relieves itching), tea tree (especially niaouli)

HERPES RELIEF

10 drops tea tree oil
5 drops myrrh oil
5 drops geranium or bergamot oil
2 drops peppermint oil (optional)
½ ounce vegetable oil

Combine the ingredients and shake or stir well. Apply directly to affected area three to five times a day during an outbreak. The peppermint oil is optional because some people find it increases rather than dulls the pain. If you would prefer a less oily formula, you can substitute either rubbing alcohol or vodka for the vegetable oil, but try a little first to make sure the alcohol doesn't sting too much.

Hives

Hives are rashlike, itchy skin bumps that are most often seen in children, but anyone can get them. They are often caused by a food allergy, although it may be difficult to diagnose at first because the reaction can occur hours or even a day after eating the culprit food. While it's a good idea to eliminate the allergen and build up the immune system, the immediate need is to stop the itching.

HIVES PASTE

¼ cup of the Hives Skin Wash (see opposite)
3 tablespoons bentonite clay (available at natural food stores)

Stir the ingredients into a paste, and wait about five minutes for it to thicken. Apply to irritated skin with your fingers or a wooden tongue depressor. Let dry on skin, and leave for at least 45 minutes before washing off. Reapply for another 30 minutes if the area is still itching.

The essential oil of chamomile is an excellent first choice to treat hives, but if it's too expensive or you don't have any on hand, you can turn to an essential oil that decreases inflammation, such as lavender. The fragrance of either lavender or chamomile oil can also be very calming to someone who feels that they are going to go mad from the itching.

First wash off the skin with a warm aromatherapy wash (see recipe below). If the itching is not sufficiently relieved, apply the Hives Paste. A child who normally objects to having a poultice smeared on his or her skin will often accept this poultice because it so effectively stops the itching.

Essential oils for hives: chamomile, lavender, peppermint

HIVES SKIN WASH

5 drops chamomile or 10 drops lavender oil
2 drops peppermint oil
3 tablespoons baking soda
2 cups water (or use peppermint tea instead)

Combine the ingredients. If you are making a tea to use as the base instead of water, pour 2½ cups of boiling water over 4 teaspoons of dried peppermint leaves, and steep 15 minutes. Strain out the herb. Add the remaining ingredients. Use a soft cloth or a skin sponge to apply on irritated skin until itching is alleviated. Chamomile is the best choice for this recipe, but it is expensive, so 10 drops of lavender essential oil can be substituted, if necessary.

Immune System, Weakened

Many essential oils have a remarkable ability to both support the immune system and increase one's rate of healing. Some of these same essential oils are also powerful antiseptics. One way these oils fight infection is to stimulate the production of white corpuscles, which are part of the body's immune defense. Still other essential oils encourage new cell growth to promote faster healing. As an extra bonus, the regenerative properties of these essential oils improve the condition and tone of the skin. All can be used in conjunction with herbal remedies designed to improve immunity. Relaxation achieved through a massage or bath lowers stress, improves sleep, and thus stimulates the immune system. (See also the section on Stress on pages 231–233 for additional treatments that can be part of your immune therapy.)

One important way to assist your immune system is with a lymphatic massage that uses essential oils. Lymph nodes are located around the body, particularly in the throat, groin, breasts, and under the arms. They are like filtering centers for cleansing the blood. The lymphatic system moves cellular fluid through the system, cleansing the body of waste produced by the body's metabolic functions. Lemon, rosemary, and grapefruit are especially good at stimulating movement and supporting the cleansing action. A lymphatic massage involves deep strokes that work from the extremities toward the heart. You can even do this on yourself. Rub the oil up your arms to the lymph nodes in your armpits. From the center of your chest, rub again toward the armpit, and then down your neck. Massage your legs from your feet up to the groin.

Essential oils for the immune system: bergamot, grapefruit, lavender, lemon, myrrh, rosemary, tea tree, thyme

IMMUNE TONIC BLEND

6 drops lavender oil
6 drops bergamot oil
3 drops lemon oil
3 drops tea tree oil
2 drops myrrh oil (expensive, so optional)
2 ounces vegetable oil

Combine ingredients. Use as a general massage oil or over specific areas of the body that tend to develop physical problems. For example, if you come down with a lot of chest colds and flus, rub this blend over your chest. Use 1 to 2 teaspoons in a bath or 1 teaspoon in a foot bath. Without the vegetable oil, this recipe is suitable for use in an aromatherapy diffuser, simmering pan of water, or potpourri cooker. Use in some form several times a day when trying to build up your own natural immunity.

LYMPH MASSAGE OIL

6 drops lemon oil
6 drops grapefruit oil
3 drops rosemary oil
2 drops bay laurel (if available)
2 ounces vegetable oil

Combine ingredients. You can use this for any type of massage, but it is particularly effective when used in a lymphatic massage as described above. It's important to use true bay laurel, sold under its botanical name *Laurus nobilis,* rather than the pimento bay that is typically sold as bay.

Indigestion/Nausea

Digestive woes such as belching, stomach pains, and intestinal gas are easily remedied with aromatherapy. A massage oil rubbed on the stomach is especially good for fussy children or anyone who refuses to swallow medicine.

Don't overlook the role that stress plays in impairing digestion. It can restrict the flow of digestive juices and constrict muscles in the digestive tract. No wonder so many people get a queasy stomach when encountering stressful situations. Tension is also thought to contribute to digestive complaints such as colitis and ulcers and most other digestive tract problems.

Aromatics start working at the first stage of digestion, when they signal the brain that food is coming. The response is almost immediate: Digestive juices are released in the mouth, stomach, and small intestine, preparing the way for proper assimilation. To aid digestion, add spices such as anise, basil, caraway, coriander, and fennel to your cooking, or drink a cup of peppermint, thyme, lemon balm, or chamomile tea. Even though many herb books describe these herbs as digestive stimulants, researchers found that most of them actually relax intestinal muscles and relieve cramping. This slower pace gives food more time to be adequately digested and, therefore, prevents gas. Thus, the same essential oils that improve poor appetite also relieve intestinal gas. These include peppermint, ginger, fennel, coriander, and dill.

Some oils have specialties: Rosemary improves poor food absorption and peppermint treats irritable bowel syndrome. Basil overcomes nausea from chemotherapy or radiation treatments (even when conventional antinausea drugs have little effect). Lemongrass is used in Brazil, the Caribbean, and much of South East Asia to relieve nervous digestion.

Essential oils for improved digestion and to eliminate gas: black pepper, clary sage, juniper berry, lemongrass, peppermint, rosemary, thyme

Essential oil to ease heartburn and stomach pain: chamomile

TUMMY OIL

2 drops lemongrass oil
1 drop fennel oil
2 drops chamomile oil
2 ounces vegetable oil

Combine the ingredients and massage over the abdominal area. This all-purpose formula will thwart indigestion, including nausea, gas, appetite loss, and motion sickness, as well as help improve appetite and digestion. You can also add 1 to 2 teaspoons to bathwater. Use as needed. Feel free to alter this formula by choosing other oils on the list, but be careful of hot oils like thyme, peppermint, and black pepper, especially in a bath since they can burn the skin.

Insect Bites

For mosquito or other insect bites that don't demand much attention, a simple dab of essential oil of lavender or tea tree provides relief from itching. Chamomile and lavender essential oils reduce swelling and inflammation, and diminish itching or other allergic response. Bentonite clay (available at your natural food store) poultices are of great help for more painful stings or bites. As the clay dries, it pulls toxins to the skin's surface to keep them from spreading, and it pulls out pus or stingers imbedded in the skin. Adding essential oil to clay keeps the clay reconstituted, preserved, and ready for an emergency. If an allergic reaction, such as excessive itching, swelling and inflammation, or difficulty breathing, occurs following a bite, call a doctor immediately.

Essential oils for bites and stings: lavender, tea tree, chamomile, peppermint (stops itching)

Essential oils that are insect repellents: birch, cedarwood, cinnamon, clove, eucalyptus, lavender, lemongrass (or citronella), orange, patchouli, peppermint (repels ants), pine, sandalwood

---

BUG-OFF REPELLENT

12 drops citronella oil
12 drops eucalyptus oil
6 drops cedarwood oil
6 drops geranium oil
1 ounce rubbing alcohol or vodka

Mix ingredients together, and dab on exposed skin. This recipe contains a lot of essential oil and is highly concentrated, so don't use it like a massage oil. Rubbing alcohol is poisonous if drunk, so if you use it, be sure to mark the container accordingly. Pat on as needed. Since it won't harm fabrics (except silk), use some of it on your clothes so that you won't apply too much to your skin or absorb too much through the skin.

BITE & STING POULTICE

12 drops lavender oil
5 drops chamomile oil
1 tablespoon bentonite clay
1 teaspoon tincture
2 teaspoons distilled water

Put clay in the container to be stored. Add the tincture and water slowly, stirring more in as the clay absorbs them. Add essential oils, stirring to distribute them evenly. The resulting mixture should be a thick paste. If necessary, add more distilled water to achieve this consistency. Store the paste in a container with a tight lid to slow dehydration. It should last several months, but if the mixture starts to dry out, add a little distilled water to reconstitute it. Use as much and as often as needed.

Insomnia

Lack of sleep is a problem for millions of Americans. Feeling tired is only one of its difficulties. Sleep deprivation can eventually lead to chronic agitation, depression, dizziness, and headaches. Once you begin to get a good night's sleep, it's possible that most of these will clear up. For general soothing and relaxation, try jasmine or marjoram. For insomnia due to mental agitation or overwork, try clary sage or rose.

One of the most relaxing treatments for children — or anyone — before bed is a warm lavender and chamomile essential oil bath. For complete relaxation, follow the bath with an aromatherapy massage. Even a simple back or foot rub often does the trick.

ZZZZ FORMULA

15 drops bergamot oil
10 drops lavender oil
10 drops sandalwood oil
3 drops frankincense (expensive, so optional)
2 drops ylang ylang oil
4 ounces vegetable oil

Combine the ingredients and use as a massage oil, or put 2 teaspoons in your bath. Feeling extravagant? Then add 2 drops of your choice of an expensive essential oil such as jasmine or rose. Without the vegetable oil, this recipe is suitable for use in an aromatherapy diffuser, simmering pan of water, or potpourri cooker. Treat yourself every night before bed as a surefire way to drift sweetly off to the Land of Nod.

You can also send children off to dreamland with a "dilly pillow." This is a small herb-filled pillow of lavender, hops, melissa, chamomile, and dill. European children used to regularly sleep with these pillows, while adults often slept on pillows stuffed simply with dried hops. Unlike most herbs, hops actually gets better with age, since exposure to air increases its sedative effects. So you don't have to worry about it losing potency if you keep it in a pillowcase!

HOPS SLEEP PILLOW

¼ cup hops strobiles
⅛ cup chamomile flowers
⅛ cup lavender flowers (optional)
⅛ cup dill weed (optional)
2 pieces of material about eight inches square

Sew material together around the edge, leaving enough room to insert a tablespoon. Fold over so stitching is inside. Combine the dried herbs and spoon them into the pillow. Sew up the opening. Lay the hops pillow under your regular sleeping pillow. If you are feeling creative, you can make the pillow any shape or size. Just make more of this recipe to fill it. A drop or two of the essential oils of lavender, chamomile, or dill can be added periodically to the fabric to refresh the scent.

Essential oils for insomnia: bergamot, chamomile, clary sage, frankincense, jasmine, lavender, marjoram, rose, sandalwood, ylang ylang

Joint Pain

A liniment heats the skin and underlying muscles and joints to relieve pain. The base of a liniment may be either rubbing alcohol or an edible alcohol such as vodka. If you do use rubbing alcohol, remember that it is toxic to drink, so label it accordingly. Alcohol is cooling and quickly evaporates, leaving no oily residue. Occasionally, though, a person will prefer using a vegetable oil base, making the liniment more like a concentrated massage oil. Oil heats up faster and will stay on the skin longer, making it better for massages.

Essential oils such as cinnamon, peppermint, and clove give a liniment its heating action. All skin-heating preparations, including Tiger Balm and White Flower Oil, contain peppermint and/or camphor, which stimulate both hot and cold reactions in nerve endings in the skin. The brain registers these sensations at the same time. The contrast between the two messages makes a liniment seem much hotter than it really is.

The most effective liniments also contain muscle-relaxing and inflammation-reducing essential oils such as rosemary, marjoram, and lavender. They penetrate into the skin to work directly on the muscle.

For arthritis, rheumatism, and other inflammatory conditions, use chamomile, marjoram, birch, and ginger in a massage oil. These same oils can also be added to a pain-relieving bath.

For arthritic hands or feet, try a daily hand or foot bath.

Essential oils for joint pain: birch, chamomile, clove, cypress, fir, ginger, juniper berry, marjoram, peppermint, rosemary

Essential oils for heating liniments: cinnamon, clove, eucalyptus, peppermint

LINIMENT

8 drops eucalyptus oil
8 drops peppermint oil
8 drops rosemary oil
4 drops cinnamon leaf oil
4 drops juniper berry oil
4 drops marjoram oil
2 ounces alcohol (either rubbing or vodka)

Mix ingredients. Shake or stir a few times daily for three days to disperse the essential oils in the alcohol. This formula is stronger than a typical massage oil, so don't use it over a large area of the body. Instead, concentrate on painful joints. It will also work well as a warm-up liniment before exercising or heavy physical work to help prevent muscles from cramping or becoming stiff (see Muscle Cramps, pages 220–222). If preferred, the alcohol in this recipe can be replaced with a vegetable oil. Use several times a day as needed.

Memory

Researchers have learned that memory recall at least doubles when a past event is associated with a smell. That's why a whiff of a fragrance can send you back in time and carry with it images and feelings associated with that event. Next time you need help accessing some elusive fact, aromatherapy can trigger your memory. Rosemary, for instance, has a long history of increasing memory, concentration, and even creativity. And modern Japanese research confirms rosemary is a brain stimulant. Other mental stimulants are sage, basil, and bay laurel.

Inhale one of the recommended essential oils while you are studying for a test or attending a class. Then, when you need to recall the information, simply smell the same scent.

Essential oils for memory: rosemary, clary sage

MEMORY FORMULA

10 drops rosemary oil
6 drops lemon oil
1 drop clary sage oil
2 ounces distilled water

Combine ingredients, and use as a spray. Without water, this formula can be used in an aromatherapy diffuser or dabbed on a tissue to smell while you are studying. The lemon oil provides both alertness and a pleasing scent.

Menopause

Not all women experience problems at menopause. But those who do will find aromatherapy at least part of the answer to them. Ideally it will be used in combination with a complete herbal program. Menopause symptoms include hot flashes, bone fragility, confusion, depression, and a dry, less elastic vagina with a thinner lining—all thought to be caused by the erratic activity or insufficiency of hormones. Several essential oils that contain hormonelike substances related to estrogen are helpful during menopause. These include clary sage, anise, fennel, cypress, angelica, coriander, sage, and to a lesser degree, basil. Such essential oils, along with peppermint and lemon, will help relieve hot flashes. Since essential oils go right through the skin, applying them to fatty areas of the body where hormones are manufactured and stored will create the most direct effect. Of course, any massage is itself very therapeutic. A bath is also a wonderful way to receive the benefits of these oils.

Geranium, neroli, and lavender are balance hormones and also help modify menopausal symptoms. They are traditionally used in European face creams to reduce aging and wrinkles. As a rejuvenation cream, these oils not only perk up a dry complexion, they make a good cream to counter vaginal dryness. Add some vitamin E oil, which improves the strength and flexibility of the vaginal lining while quickly healing abrasions that can occur during intercourse when the lining is too dry. In addition to aromatherapy, try dietary and herbal treatments to alleviate some of menopause's unpleasant symptoms.

Essential oils that affect estrogen and balance hormones: cypress, geranium, lavender, neroli, rose, clary sage

Essential oils that ease hot flashes: clary sage, lemon, peppermint

Essential oils for emotional ups and downs: chamomile, jasmine, neroli

MENOPAUSE BODY OIL

6 drops lemon oil
5 drops geranium oil
2 drops clary sage oil
1 drop angelica oil
1 drop jasmine oil
2 ounces vegetable oil or body lotion

Combine the ingredients. Use at least once a day as a massage oil, in a lotion, or in a bath (add 2 teaspoons to the bathwater). If this formula is too oily for you, add the same essential oils to 2 ounces of a commercial body lotion instead. The best type to use is an unscented, basic lotion that contains ingredients that are as natural as possible.

Rejuvenation Oil

6 drops geranium oil
6 drops lavender
1 drop neroli
1500 units vitamin E oil
1 ounce vegetable oil

Combine ingredients. For the vitamin E, either buy the liquid vitamin or open vitamin capsules and empty the contents into your preparation. Apply to both the inside and outside of the vagina as needed. You can also stir these essential oils into a prepared cream.

Muscle Cramps

Muscles can hurt after a vigorous day of exercise or work, especially if you aren't exercising on a regular basis and then really go for it. Activities that you repeat daily can also tighten muscles and cause them to cramp. The oil formula below is excellent for lower back or shoulder pain, tight muscles from working at a computer, or the aftereffects of physical exercise. Even menstrual cramps, which are really little more than the cramping of the uterine muscle, respond well to this remedy. By the way, this same recipe can be used as a first-aid treatment along with ice on sprains and bruises. The sooner it is applied, the better. It reduces the swelling and pain and promotes faster healing.

The latest medical thinking is that you should use a liniment containing heating oils to increase blood circulation and warmth to an area before exercising rather than waiting until afterward. By doing so, the liniment works like a mini warm-up for the muscles. You'll still want to do your warm-up exercises, but the combination will give you extra warmth, helping to prevent muscle cramps. See Joint Pain, pages 215–216, for more on liniments and for an aromatherapy liniment recipe. Then, if your muscles do cramp, use the cramp relief oil below to relax them.

CRAMP RELIEF OIL

12 drops lavender oil
6 drops marjoram oil
4 drops chamomile oil
4 drops ginger oil
2 ounces vegetable oil or St. John's wort oil

Combine ingredients. Apply throughout the day as often as needed over the cramping area. This formula is also excellent for the lower back pain that sometimes accompanies menstrual cramps. It works well when made with plain vegetable oil, but if you can, use an herbal oil made from St. John's wort oil instead, as it is excellent for sore muscles. You can buy a ready-made version at natural food stores.

Essential oils for muscle pains and menstrual cramps: birch, chamomile, ginger, jasmine, lavender, marjoram, melissa, rosemary

Nausea/Motion Sickness

That queasy feeling in the stomach that signals nausea can be caused by quite a few different problems. Topping the list are motion sickness, food poisoning, the flu, headaches, emotional upset, anxiety, medications, and pregnancy. Peppermint and ginger ease both nausea and motion sickness. Chamomile and fennel relax the stomach and soothe burning irritation and inflammation. Basil overcomes nausea from chemotherapy or radiation treatments (even when conventional antinausea drugs have little effect). Lemongrass is used in Brazil, the Caribbean, and much of South East Asia to relieve nervous digestion. Sometimes the smell alone of such essential oils as peppermint, ginger, or basil is enough to quell nausea. If not, use them in a massage oil where they will enter the bloodstream.

Prefer the taste of peppermint? It comes in a close second in preventing motion sickness and works equally well for general stomach upsets. While essential oils are far too potent to ingest, you can take the extract of peppermint that is sold at the grocery store in the baking section. Used mostly to flavor candy, this product is a diluted and water soluble form of the essential oil. A couple drops of peppermint extract in a glass of water makes a handy first aid remedy. If you are prone to motion sickness, carry a small vial of the extract with you on your next airplane flight, boat ride, or any form of travel.

Essential oils for nausea and motion sickness: ginger, peppermint, sandalwood

---

STOMACH SOOTHER

*1–3 drops peppermint extract
(not in essential oil form!)
½–1 cup water (preferably warm)*

Add the extract to the water. Sip to ease nausea or stomach upset, and repeat after 20–30 minutes if you haven't experienced relief.

Nerve Pain

The nerves in your body register pain, so when nerves are damaged, the condition will be quite painful. Injured nerves take a long time to regenerate, but aromatherapy treatments can help with the process. They initially relieve pain, and people who use them appear to heal more quickly than others.

Essential oils of lavender, chamomile, and marjoram are excellent at easing the pain of a pinched nerve or sciatica. A less well-known essential oil called helichrysum is specific for this condition. Apply the oil directly on the back or hip to reduce pain. It is also wonderful on painful shingles. People with serious nerve-related problems, such as multiple sclerosis and chronic fatigue syndrome, get noticeable pain relief from the Nerve Pain Oil (see recipe below). For carpal tunnel syndrome, rub this oil into the wrists. Since nerve conditions can be difficult to heal, talk to someone skilled in natural medicine for more ideas on how to treat them.

Essential oils for nerve pain: chamomile, lavender, marjoram, peppermint, sandalwood

---

NERVE PAIN OIL

4 drops chamomile oil
3 drops marjoram oil
3 drops helichrysum oil (if available)
2 drops lavender oil
1 ounce vegetable oil or St. John's wort oil

Combine the ingredients. Apply as needed throughout the day for pain relief. This formula is even more effective if St. John's wort oil is used instead of plain vegetable oil. Buy it at a natural food store.

Poison Oak/Ivy/Sumac

The infamous, extremely itchy rash that is caused by touching poison oak or poison ivy is a type of dermatitis that calls for special aromatherapy care. Use a vinegar base, as oil-based products aren't usually recommended in the first stages. However, some people find that a lotion relieves the later dry stage.

OAT BATH

3 drops of any oil from the list
1 drop peppermint oil
4 cups quick-cooking oats (they dissolve best)
1 cup Epsom salts
a square of muslin or double-layered cheesecloth

Add the essential oils to the oats and put them into the cloth, which should be tied to form a bag. Put all ingredients in a lukewarm bath and soak yourself in it. Do this several times a day if it helps. Or mix a smaller amount of oats dissolved in hot water with the essential oils, and sponge it on.

Choose essential oils that slow the inflammation and ease the itching. Peppermint may seem an unlikely essential oil to use, but the menthol it contains relieves the painful burning and itching that accompany the rash.

If you can, first soak the affected area in a tepid oatmeal bath such as the one suggested above. Then apply the remedy described on page 226. Some people find that even warm water is irritating, so experiment with water temperature to find what works best for you.

Essential oils for poison oak/ivy/sumac: chamomile, cypress, geranium, lavender, peppermint

POISON OAK/IVY/SUMAC REMEDY

3 drops lavender oil
3 drops cypress oil
3 drops peppermint oil
½ teaspoon salt
1 tablespoon warm water
1 tablespoon apple cider vinegar
1 ounce calendula tincture

Dissolve the salt in the water and vinegar; then add the other ingredients. Shake well to disperse and again before each use. Apply externally as needed to the rash.

Premenstrual Syndrome (PMS)

Premenstrual syndrome, better known as PMS, is a collection of many different symptoms that typically begin several days or even a week before menstruation. The host of symptoms include water retention, breast swelling and tenderness, depression, irritability, mood swings, and headaches. Not all women who get PMS experience all of these symptoms, but any one of them can greatly alter one's life while going through it.

In many ways, aromatherapy is ideal to treat PMS. Taking time out to lounge in an aromatic bath or getting a massage with a fragrant oil helps most women tremendously. For depression and mood swings associated with PMS, nothing can beat clary sage. The essential oils of neroli, rose, and jasmine may be expensive, but their heavenly fragrances help dispel moodiness and irritability.

For the excessive bloating and swollen breasts of PMS, use the essential oils of juniper berry, patchouli, grapefruit, and carrot seed. Another good oil for this is birch, which is also a natural

MOOD OIL

9 drops geranium oil
6 drops chamomile oil
3 drops clary sage oil
3 drops angelica oil (optional)
2 drops marjoram oil
2 ounces vegetable oil

Combine the ingredients. The angelica oil is heavenly, but optional, as it may be hard to find. Use daily as a massage oil or add 1 to 2 teaspoons to a bath. This recipe improves your mood even if you don't have PMS. To make it more elegant and effective, add 1 or 2 drops of neroli, rose, or jasmine. Without the vegetable oil, you can use this in a diffuser or simply carry around a vial of it to smell as needed.

pain reliever. Use juniper berry if you experience water retention. If headache is among your PMS symptoms, try an inhalation of lavender or marjoram. For best results with any PMS or menstruation remedy, begin using it a couple of days before you experience any symptoms. Refer also to the sections on fatigue, acne, and menstrual cramps.

Essential oils for PMS: chamomile, clary sage, geranium, jasmine, marjoram, neroli, rose

Essential oils for bloating: birch, juniper berry, lavender, patchouli

BLOATING AND HEADACHE RELIEF OIL

6 drops lavender oil
3 drops juniper berry oil
2 drops birch oil
1 drop patchouli oil (optional)

Combine ingredients. Use as a massage oil or add 1 to 2 teaspoons to your bath or 1 teaspoon to a foot bath. Don't use the patchouli if you don't like the smell; it can easily overwhelm a formula.

Sore Throat/Laryngitis

A bacterial infection or lots of singing, talking, or yelling can cause a sore throat. At times, the throat can be so inflamed and painful that it becomes difficult to swallow. If the inflammation is in the voice box, you can easily come down with laryngitis, in which your voice is reduced to a hoarse whisper or it even may become impossible to talk at all.

For centuries, European singers have known the secret to preserving their voices with aromatherapy and herbal remedies. Their most popular sore throat and laryngitis cure is to gargle with a marjoram herb tea that has been sweetened with honey. You can use the essential oil of marjoram to make a similar remedy. As both an antiseptic and anti-inflammatory, it is a good choice. Other essential oils or herb teas to use as a gargle are sage, hyssop, and thyme, all of which kill bacterial infections.

Any of these essential oils can easily be gargled or sprayed into the throat. This brings the antibacterial and soothing essential oils into direct contact with the bacteria responsible for causing a sore throat or laryngitis. In an emergency, a few drops of essential oil diluted in two ounces of water may also be used. In addition, try a neck wrap as given on page 229. This is especially good to use if your glands are swollen or your neck is stiff.

Both lavender and eucalyptus work so well in an aromatherapy steam to recover your voice that you must remind yourself to not overstress it until your throat fully recovers. And don't forget the old standard of a hot drink made with fresh lemon juice and honey.

Essential oils for sore throat: bergamot, eucalyptus, lavender, lemon, marjoram, sage, sandalwood, tea tree, thyme

THROAT SPRAY OR GARGLE

4 drops marjoram oil
½ cup warm water
½ teaspoon salt

Combine ingredients. Shake well to dissolve
the salt and disperse the oils before spraying or
gargling. Gargle every half hour at first and
then several times a day.

NECK WRAP

2 drops lavender oil
2 drops bergamot oil
1 drop tea tree oil
2 cups hot water

Mix the water with the essential oils. While
still warm, soak a soft cloth, preferably flannel,
in the water and wring it out. Wrap it around
the neck. Cover with a towel (thin enough to
be comfortable) to hold in the heat. Remove
before it becomes cold. Use throughout the
day as often as you wish.

Stress

Stress is part of life. It has a powerful effect on the body and takes its toll on both mental and physical well-being. It can cause headaches, nervous indigestion, or heart palpitations. Medical research now says that stress may be largely responsible for causing or at least promoting more serious disorders such as heart disease and allergies. Stress also overworks the adrenal glands. Repeated release of an overabundance of adrenaline from these glands eventually disrupts the delicate balance of your brain chemistry and hormonal production. Initially this will make you feel like you are always on edge. Eventually, the adrenal glands become exhausted and the opposite reaction occurs. You become tired, sluggish, listless, and emotions may easily fly out of control.

It is not always easy to avoid stress, but there are ways you can cope with it better. Fortunately, aromatherapy offers some of the best types of natural prescriptions for easing stress. There are many relaxing fragrances listed on the next page. For starters, incorporate these scents into your life in as many ways as possible, especially by using the ideas and recipes given throughout this book.

When applying the oil formulas, give yourself several minutes of slow, deep, even breathing while you imagine how, with each breath, the oil molecules are entering your bloodstream, and spreading throughout your body, relaxing tight muscles and alleviating tensions and strain. These moments will soon become one of your favorite times of the day.

Lavender, bergamot, marjoram, sandalwood, lemon, and chamomile were found (in that order) to relax brain waves. Doctors Giovanni Gatti and Renato Cayola discovered that the most sedating oils for their patients were neroli, petitgrain, chamomile, valerian, and opopanax (which is similar to myrrh). In fact, neroli, valerian, and nutmeg are included in a blend patented by International Flavors and Fragrances, Inc., for easing stress in the workplace. Aromatherapists find ylang ylang another potent relaxant. Need evenmore ways to relax? See Insomnia, pages 212–214.

Essential oils that relax and sedate: bergamot, chamomile, lavender, lemon, marjoram, neroli, orange, sandalwood, ylang ylang

RELAXING BATH

2 drops bergamot oil
1 drop petitgrain oil

Add oils directly to the bath and stir to distribute. See "Application Formulas" for additional ways to create a soothing bath. You can enjoy this bath daily.

Relaxing Massage Oil

10 drops lavender oil
6 drops chamomile oil
4 drops ylang ylang oil
4 drops sandalwood oil (expensive, so optional)
2 ounces vegetable oil

Combine ingredients. Use as a massage oil as needed, or add 1 or 2 teaspoons to your bath or 1 teaspoon to a footbath. To add sophistication and an extra lift to this blend, add 1 drop of neroli essential oil. For children less than 8 years of age, use half the quantity of essential oil recommended. Without the vegetable oil, this combination can be used in an aromatherapy diffuser, simmering pan of water, or a potpourri cooker, or you can add it to 2 ounces of water for an air spray. Use daily and as often as you like.

Toothache

For more than a century, clove bud oil has been used to ease all types of tooth pain, at least until you can get to the dentist. Even dentists themselves still recommend clove oil to their patients, and it is found in several dental preparations. Use the essential oil that is made from the bud instead of the leaf because the leaf contains so much of the constituent eugenol that it is considered somewhat toxic. In an emergency, put a clove bud in your mouth where it hurts the most. As it softens, mash the clove gently with your teeth to release the oil, and suck on it.

To relieve teething pain, rub the child's gums with a little Toothache Oil on your finger. Clove bud oil can be hot, so try it in your own mouth first. If it is still too hot, dilute it with more vegetable oil before putting it in your baby's month.

Essential oils for toothache: chamomile, clove

TOOTHACHE OIL

4 drops clove bud oil
1 drop orange oil (for flavor)
1 teaspoon vegetable oil

Combine ingredients. Rub a few drops onto painful gums. Repeat every half hour or so. If your child refuses the clove teething oil, try replacing the clove oil with chamomile oil. The chamomile is a less effective pain reliever, but it isn't hot like the clove. Apply the treatment several times a day, as needed

---

Uterine Problems

There are a variety of uterine problems, including endometriosis, pelvic inflammatory disease, cervical dysplasia, and serious menstrual cramps, for which aromatherapy is useful as an adjunct to other treatments. Endometriosis is a displacement of the uterine lining on the outside of the uterus or other areas where it doesn't belong. This condition causes inflammation and scarring and can be very painful. Pelvic inflammatory disease, nicknamed PID, is a very serious problem because it is usually a result of a difficult-to-treat infection in the uterine tissue. Cervical dysplasia is precancerous cell growth on the cervix. Menstrual cramps are muscle cramping that occurs in the uterus during menstruation; for some women, the cramps are so painful that they are debilitating. For more about muscle relaxation and pain, see Menstrual Cramps, pages 220–222.

A massage oil made from relaxing essential oils like lavender and chamomile helps relieve the inflammation, discomfort, and even the pain of most uterine problems. Rosemary promotes circulation.

Two treatments handy for encouraging uterine healing are the castor oil pack and the sitz bath combined with aromatherapy. No one can explain exactly how these treatments work, but herbalists and aromatherapists have seen what a difference they can make.

The sitz bath requires two tubs large enough to sit in so that water covers the abdomen. It is best if these can both fit into your bathtub, where spilling water won't be a problem. Fill one with hot water and the other with cold. You can also use the bathtub for hot water and have a plastic tub next to it on the floor for cold. Switch back and forth between the hot and cold about four times. Four minutes in the hot and one minute in the cold is tolerable and actually feels good after a few rounds. You will soon want the hot hotter and the cold colder!

The sitz bath employs hot and cold water, which is a simple medical treatment used since ancient times to increase blood circulation, since the increased blood flow speeds healing by bringing nutrients to all areas of the body and spurring the removal of toxins. A recent study from Washington University in Washington, DC, found that a castor oil pack improves the action of the immune system in the pelvic area when placed on the abdomen. Instructions for the castor oil pack are on the opposite page.

Essential oils for uterine problems: chamomile, lavender, rosemary.

SITZ BATH

5 drops rosemary oil
5 drops lavender oil

Add the essential oils to the hot bath only. Sit in a tub with the hot water up to your waist for five to ten minutes. Then switch to a tub of cold water for at least one minute. The large plastic tubs sold at hardware stores work well for this. Continue for two to five rounds. Do this treatment every day, if possible, or at least twice a week.

CASTOR OIL PACK

8 drops lavender oil
¼ cup castor oil
soft cloth

Combine lavender and castor oils. Soak the cloth in oil. Fold the cloth, and place it in a baking dish in the oven set at 350°F for about 20 minutes. It should be quite warm, but not uncomfortable. Place the folded cloth directly over the uterus and cover with a towel to keep it warm. (Placing a hot water bottle or heating pad on top and surrounding it all with a towel works even better.) Afterward, rinse off the oil. Keep the pack on for 30 to 60 minutes, two or three times per week until the condition has cleared.

Varicose Veins/ Hemorrhoids

Varicose veins and hemorrhoids both occur when circulating blood slows down on its way back to the heart. Blood relies on muscles in your legs and pelvis to push it back to the heart — not an easy task if you spend your day sitting or standing for long periods. If you are very overweight, pregnant, or constipated, or if you wear skin-tight pants or a girdle, blood flow through your pelvic area is also restricted. Over time, this extra blood load causes veins to weaken and stretch, resulting in extended veins on the legs that show as blue streaks running up and down the leg or as hemorrhoids, which are dilated and protruding veins in or around the anus.

LAVENDER CARROT COMPRESS

3 drops chamomile oil
3 drops carrot seed oil
3 drops lavender oil
1 cup cold water
1 teaspoon tincture of calendula
or St. John's wort

Combine ingredients. Stir a soft cloth in the solution, wring it out, and place it over itching or broken varicose veins or hemorrhoids as often as practical. It can be used daily. The tinctures should be available at natural food stores.

There is usually little treatment outside of surgery that doctors can offer anyone who has varicose veins or hemorrhoids. However, essential oils of chamomile, palmarosa, myrtle, frankincense, and cypress reduce enlarged veins, ease the inflammation, and lessen pain. Massage oils containing these essential oils can be gently rubbed on the veins. When massaging the legs, use upward strokes that go with the blood flow, and be sure you don't push too deeply since these veins are already fragile.

VEIN OIL

10 drops palmarosa oil
8 drops cypress oil
7 drops chamomile oil
1 ounce vegetable oil or St. John's wort oil

Combine ingredients. Apply externally directly over problem area (as described above) one or two times a day. This recipe works best when added to an infused oil of St. John's wort, which you can buy in natural food stores.

If varicose veins and hemorrhoids reach the point at which the skin breaks and ulcers form, apply a compress of lavender essential oil. Carrot seed essential oil specifically helps conditions where there is inflammation associated with enlarged veins, although it can be difficult to find and may need to be special ordered.

Essential oils for varicose veins: chamomile, cypress, frankincense, juniper berry, lavender, myrrh

Warts

Warts are raised areas on the skin that are often bumpy and dark in color. Genital warts are caused by the human papilloma virus (HPV). Difficult to detect, genital warts will temporarily turn whitish if you dab on vinegar that has been diluted in an equal amount of water.

Tea tree and particularly thuja essential oils are two of the most effective wart removers. Thuja is very strong, so use it carefully. Essential oils often get rid of warts, although the virus does stay in the system and can pop out again. For some reason, the aromatherapy treatment works in some cases, but not in others.

Essential oils for warts: tea tree, thuja

WART OIL

12 drops tea tree oil
12 drops thuja oil
1 teaspoon castor oil or vegetable oil
800 IU vitamin E oil

Combine the ingredients. Apply directly to the wart(s) two to four times daily. Castor oil is a good choice of vegetable oil since it is a folk treatment for warts. Adding vitamin E facilitates healing. It can be obtained by pricking two 400 IU capsules with a pin and squeezing out the contents. This is a high concentration of essential oil, and thuja is particularly strong, so use a glass rod applicator, dropper, or cotton swab to apply and be sure not to get it on the skin around the wart since repeated use can burn sensitive skin.

RESOURCES

ORGANIZATIONS AND NEWSLETTERS

American Alliance of Aromatherapy
(800) 809-9850
Newsletter: *News Quarterly*
Distributes: *International Journal of Aromatherapy*

American Herb Association
P.O. Box 1673
Nevada City, CA 95959
(916) 265-9552
Newsletter: *AHA Quarterly*
Includes herbs & aromatherapy.
Offers:
AHA *Directory of Mail Order Herbal & Aromatherapy Products* $4.
AHA *Directory of Herbal Education* (Includes aromatherapy) $3.50.

Aromatic Thymes
18-4 East Dundee Rd., Suite 200
Barrington, IL 60010
(847) 526-0456

Aromatherapy Quarterly (US)
P.O. Box 421
Inverness, CA 94937
(415) 663-9519
E-mail: aromamag@nbn.com

National Association for Holistic Aromatherapy
(NAHA)
P.O. Box 17622
Boulder, CO 80308
Newsletter: *Scentsitivity*
Local chapters throughout US
(888) ASK-NAHA (toll free)
E-mail: info@naha.org
Website: http://www.naha.org

Canadian & English Associations

Aromatherapy World
ISPA House, 82 Ashby Rd.
Hinckley, Leics
England, LEIO ISN

Canadian Federation of Aromatherapists
Box 68571-1235 Williams Pky. East
Brampton, Ontario L6S 6A1
Newsletter: *Escential News*

International Federation of Aromatherapists
Stamford House
2-4 Chiswick High Rd.
London, England W4 1TH

International Society for Professional Aromatherapists
ISPA House, 82 Ashby Rd.
Hinckley, Leics LE10 1SN

Register of Qualified Aromatherapists
Box 66941
London, England N8 9HF

The Tisserand Institute
6 Church Rd,
Hoye, East Sussex
England BNI 3PY
Newsletter: *International Journal of Aromatherapy*

Professional Associations & Journals

The Journal of Essential Oil Research. Allured Publishing
Corp. 362 S. Schmale Rd., Carol Stream, IL 60188.
(630) 653-2155.

Perfumer & Flavorist. Allured Publishing Corp. 362 S.
Schmale Rd., Carol Stream, IL 60188. (630) 653-2155

US Essential Oil Trade. 1993 Publication. Circular Series,
US Department of Agriculture, Foreign Agricultural
Service, Room 4655-S, Washington, DC 20250-1000.

The Flavor & Extract Manufacturer's Association of the
United States. FEMA, 500 C Street, SW, Washington,
DC 20006. (202) 646-2400

Mail order essential oils & products

Aroma Land
1326 Rufina Circle
Santa Fe, NM 87505
(800) 933-5267
Aroma jewelry & lamps

Aromatherapy Trades Council
P.O. Box 38, Romford,
Essex, England RMI 2DN
(Provides list of suppliers)

Leydet Aromatics
P.O. Box 2354
Fair Oaks, CA 95628
Aromatherapy seminars

Oak Valley Herb Farm
Kathi Keville
P.O. Box 2482
Nevada City, CA 95959
(530) 274-3140
Essential oils, aromatherapy massage bath & body oils,
cosmetics, herbal products
Catalog $1

Original Swiss Aromatics
P.O. Box 606
San Rafael, CA 94915
Essential oils, base ingredients, cosmetics
Catalog: $1

Prima Fleur Botanicals
1201-R Anderson Dr.
San Rafael, CA 94901
(415) 455-0956
Essential oils

Simpler's Botanical Co.
P.O. Box 39
Forestville, CA 95436
Hydrosols, essential oils, carrier oils, herbal extracts,
cosmetics

INDEX

A

Abies alba. See Fir.
Abies balsamea. See Fir.
Abies siberica. See Fir.
Abscesses, 127
Absolutes, 49
Absorption, of oils, 39
Acetic acid, 141
Acetic esters, 143
Acids, 43
Acne,
  aromatic waters for, 76
  essential oils for, 102, 108, 115,
    120, 122, 129, 134, 137, 157,
    159
  treatments, 170–172
Agarwood, 26
Aging, 143, 153, 189, 190
Air fresheners. See Diffusers; Room
  sprays.
Alcohols
  carriers, 63–64
  in ginger, 124
  in liniments, 74, 215
  medicinal properties, 42
Aldehydes, 38, 42, 145
Alexander the Great, 10–11
Allergic reactions, 104
Allspice, 92
Aloe vera, 177
Alpha androsterole, 156
Alpha pinene, 164
Alpha terpineol, 127
Alzheimer disease, 41
Amarakinon, 19
Amber, 26
Ambergris, 23
Angelica, 29, 43, 195, 218
Anise, 25, 83, 179, 209, 218
Anthemis nobilis. See Roman
  chamomile.

Antibacterials, 95, 110, 114, 117,
  141, 153, 159, 161. *See also*
  Bacterial infections.
Antibiotics, 97
Antihistamines, 110
Antioxidants, 95, 139, 155, 161
Antiseptics, 92, 97, 100, 102, 104,
  106, 112, 119, 122, 129, 131,
  133, 136, 141, 148, 153, 155,
  157, 160–161
Anxiety, 41, 45, 97, 145, 164,
  184–185
Aphrodisiacs, 8, 105, 109, 124, 127,
  148, 150, 156, 163
Appetite stimulants, 103, 105, 124,
  155, 209
Appetite suppressants, 148
Aqua Mirabilis (Miracle Water), 29,
  30
Aromacology, defined, 44
Aroma notes, 67
Aromatherapy
  defined, 34–35
  history, 6–7
  term coined, 32
Aromatic compounds, 37–39, 42–43
Aromatic waters, 7, 28–30, 76–77
Arthritis, 100, 110, 114, 129,
  215–216
Aspirin, natural, 99
Association, and sense of smell,
  41–44
Asthma, 108, 115, 117, 153, 173–175
Astringents, 100, 102, 108, 112, 119,
  122, 129, 136, 141, 153, 155,
  157, 161
Athlete's foot, 110, 141, 148,
  195–198
Attar of roses, 152
Augustus, Emperor, 13
Azulene, 150

B

Baby oil, making, 188
Baby powder, making, 188

Methyl anthranilate, 145
Methyl salicylate, 99, 100
Migraines, 41, 131, 139, 199–200.
    See also Headaches.
Mint, 26
Miracle Water, 29, 30
Mohammed, 13
Mold, 117, 137
Mood, enhancing, 129, 145, 227
Mood swings, 45
Moses, 23
Moth repellents, 101, 128, 147. *See
    also* Insect repellents.
Motion sickness, 125, 222–223
Mouthwash, 72–73, 161–162
MQV, 158
Mucous. *See* Congestion.
Multiple sclerosis, 167, 224
Muscle cramps, 220–222
Muscle pain/stiffness, 72, 74, 78,
    100, 104, 106, 110, 115, 117,
    125, 129, 131, 155, 161
Muscle relaxants, 92, 104, 106, 108,
    112, 127, 131, 139, 143, 145,
    150, 164
Musk, 13, 26
Myrcene, 108, 129, 133, 136
Myrrh
    cautions, 85
    history, 8–10, 13, 23, 24
    profile, 140–141
    properties, 57
    uses, 182–183, 189, 196, 198, 203,
    207, 239
Myrrholic acid, 141
Myrtle, 11, 238

N

Napoleon, 30
Nasal inhalers, natural, 73, 180, 181,
    185
Nausea, 104, 125, 151, 157, 164,
    208–210, 222–223
Neat, defined, 91
Neck strain, 72

Neck wrap, 230
Nero, Emperor, 12
Nerol, 143, 153
Neroli
    history, 30
    profile, 142–143
    properties, 43
    uses, 82, 184, 189, 218, 227, 232
Nerolidol, 104, 143
Nerve pain, 150, 157, 223–224
Nerves/nervousness. *See* Mental
    relaxants.
Niaouli, 43, 158, 203. *See also* Tea
    Tree.
Nutmeg, 12, 16, 232

O

Oat bath, 225
Odor intensity, 67–68
Oily hair, 129, 137, 164
Oily skin, 112, 115, 134, 170–172
Olfaction Research Group, 45
Olibanol, 119
Opopanax, 232
Optimism, 36
Oral infections, 97, 140, 141,
    161
Orange
    blending, 68
    cautions, 79
    processing, 48, 51
    profile, 144–146
    properties, 45, 61
    storing, 57
    uses, 36, 184, 211, 232
Orange blossom. *See* Neroli.
Orange flower water, 142
Orange water, 14
Oregano, 42, 92
Oregon grape root, 162
Origanum marjorana. *See* Marjoram.
Orris root, 86
Overheating, compress for, 71
Oxides, 43

P

Pain relievers, 72, 139, 150
Palmarosa, 136, 238
Palsy Drops, 199
Pandanus, 26
Panic, 36
Paranoia, 184
Parasitic infections, 159, 161
Patchoulene, 148
Patchouli
  history, 12, 26
  profile, 147–148
  properties, 42, 57
  uses, 82, 86, 194, 202, 211, 227
Patchoulol, 148
Pearly everlasting, 18
Pelargonium graveoloens. See
  Geranium.
Pelvic inflammatory disease (PID),
  234
Pennyroyal, 42
Pepper, black, 11, 194, 209
Peppermint
  cautions, 79
  cost, 56
  processing, 51, 52
  profile, 149–151
  properties, 42, 45, 61
  uses, 44, 74, 83, 173, 178, 179,
    187, 189, 194, 195, 196, 199,
    202, 205, 209, 211, 215, 218,
    222, 224, 225
Perfume
  benzoin as fixative, 94
  birth of industry, 31–32
  derivation, 6
  houses, 31–32
  invention of, 27–32
  solid, 8, 11, 16–17, 22–23
  uses, 18–19, 82
Personality, of scent, 67
Perspiration. *See* Sweating.
Petitgrain, 42, 143, 145, 184,
  232
Pharmacological action, 34
Phellandrene, 108

Phenols, 38, 42, 131
Phenylacetic acid, 127
Phenyl ethanol, 153
Phenylethylene, 95
Phenylpropylic alcohol, 95
Photosensitivity, from oils, 98, 134,
  146
Physical disabilities, 138
Physiological action, 34
Picea species. *See* Fir.
PID. *See* Pelvic inflammatory
  disease.
Pillows, 201, 213–214
Pimples, 79. *See also* Acne.
Pine, 11, 26, 175, 194, 211
Pinene, 104, 108, 112, 114, 117, 129,
  131, 133, 141, 143, 155, 159
Pinocarvone, 104
Pinus species. *See* Fir.
Piperitone, 114
Pipettes, 60
Plague, 109
PMS, 104, 108, 122, 127, 143, 153,
  226–228
Pogostemon cablin. See Patchouli.
Pogostol, 148
Poison ivy/oak/sumac, 151, 186,
  224–226
Pomme d'ambre, 23
Pores, opening, 71
Potpourri cookers, 87–88
Potpourris, 86–87, 94
Poultices, 205, 212
Powders, making, 188, 198
Prayer, inspiring, 140
Pregnancy, and oils, 102, 108, 146,
  162
Premenstrual syndrome. *See* PMS.
Prescription drugs, 166, 184
Preservatives, 95, 139
Price, of oils, 54–56
Protection, 128
Psoriasis, 75, 100, 102, 186–187
Psychological action, 34
Pulegone, 150
Purification, 17–18, 154
Purity, of oils, 50–51